ADVANCE PRAISE FOR EMERGENCY NEUROLOGY, SECOND EDITION

"*Emergency Neurology* provides practical guidance to approaching both common as well as newly described neurological syndromes. With illustrative cases, key points, and useful tables, each chapter addresses common diagnostic and therapeutic dilemmas in a brief, engaging, and high impact format. *Emergency Neurology* is a useful resource for clinicians at all levels of training and experience in neurology."

—John Probasco, MD, Vice Chair for Quality,
Safety, and Service, Department of Neurology,
Johns Hopkins University School of Medicine,
Baltimore, Maryland

"Now more than ever, hospital neurologists must be nimble and integrative in responding to complex consultations and urgent cases as their scope of practice continues to expand rapidly. In this Second Edition of *Emergency Neurology*, LaHue and Levin offer nuanced yet pragmatic approaches filled with clinical pearls relevant to trainees and seasoned clinicians alike. This book will get you into the mindset of a modern neurohospitalist and will surely improve your practice."

—Joshua P. Klein, MD, PhD, Vice Chair, Clinical Affairs,
and Chief, Division of Hospital Neurology,
Department of Neurology, Brigham and
Women's Hospital, Boston, Massachusetts

"This book makes it easy to grasp collection of critical issues pertinent to approaching a clinic, hospitalized patient, curbside consult, morning report, or clinic conference. The text is loaded with logical, stepwise approaches to differential diagnosis, gently guiding the reader on how to proceed in the golden hours of neurological emergencies. Ample updates sprinkled throughout the text span the breadth of topics with significant advances in recent years—comprehensive, easy on the eyes, and an essential guide for every clinician."

—Vineeta Singh, MD, Professor of Neurology,
University of California, San Francisco

T0177832

What Do I Do Now?

SERIES CO-EDITORS-IN-CHIEF

Lawrence C. Newman, MD
Director of the Headache Division
Professor of Neurology
New York University Langone
New York, New York

Morris Levin, MD
Director of the Headache Center
Professor of Neurology
University of California, San Francisco
San Francisco, California

Emergency Neurology

SECOND EDITION

Sara C. LaHue, MD
Assistant Professor of Clinical Neurology
Department of Neurology
University of California
San Francisco, CA, USA

Morris Levin, MD
Professor
Department of Neurology
University of California
San Francisco, CA, USA

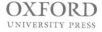
OXFORD
UNIVERSITY PRESS

OXFORD
UNIVERSITY PRESS

Oxford University Press is a department of the University of Oxford. It furthers
the University's objective of excellence in research, scholarship, and education
by publishing worldwide. Oxford is a registered trade mark of Oxford University
Press in the UK and certain other countries.

Published in the United States of America by Oxford University Press
198 Madison Avenue, New York, NY 10016, United States of America.

© Oxford University Press 2021

Library of Congress Cataloging-in-Publication Data
Names: LaHue, Sara C., author. | Levin, Morris, 1955– author.
Title: Emergency neurology / Sara C. LaHue, Morris Levin.
Other titles: What do I do now?
Description: 2nd edition. | New York, NY : Oxford University Press, [2021] |
Series: What do I do now | Morris Levin's name appears first on previous edition. |
Includes bibliographical references and index.
Identifiers: LCCN 2020020672 (print) | LCCN 2020020673 (ebook) |
ISBN 9780190064303 (paperback) | ISBN 9780190064327 (epub) |
ISBN 9780190064334 (online)
Subjects: MESH: Central Nervous System Diseases | Emergencies | Case Reports
Classification: LCC RC350.7 (print) | LCC RC350.7 (ebook) | NLM WL 301 |
DDC 616.8/0425—dc23
LC record available at https://lccn.loc.gov/2020020672
LC ebook record available at https://lccn.loc.gov/2020020673

DOI: 10.1093/med/9780190064303.001.0001

9 8 7 6 5 4 3 2
Printed by Marquis, Canada

Contents

SECTION 2 TREATMENT DILEMMAS

SECTION 3 PEDIATRIC DILEMMAS

Preface

Some of the most exciting recent developments in neurology have occurred in the management of neurologic emergencies. This case-based second edition of *Emergency Neurology* features 13 new chapters as well as significant updates to chapters that appeared in the first edition and that provide practical approaches incorporating these clinical advances. The topics include acute stroke management and stroke prevention, status epilepticus, neurologic toxicities from cancer immunotherapy, newly appreciated autoimmune and paraneoplastic diseases, the prevention and management of delirium, and many others.

"Can I tell you about a new case?" is a common refrain among medical colleagues who strive to learn from each other and from our patients. Sharing cases serves as an internal check to our personal systematic approaches to the management of various diseases and are a delightfully interactive way to stay up to date in medicine. A number of clinical presentations that we see lead to diagnostic or therapeutic impasses (i.e., "What do I do now?"). We have tried to identify important examples and sort through them in a comprehensive but practical way. Our point of view is often that of an attendee at a morning rounds discussion, starting with key details of a relevant case, followed by a pragmatic discussion of the differential diagnosis, testing options, and management strategies.

This book is for clinicians at all levels of training and in all fields of medicine who treat patients with urgent or emergent neurological illnesses. This book can serve as a reference for common clinical questions or a focused primer to prepare the busy consultant for a number of eventualities on service. We hope that sharing our passion for caring for patients suffering from neurologic emergencies deepens your knowledge and clinical practice.

Sara C. LaHue, MD
Morris Levin, MD
San Francisco, CA, USA

Acknowledgments

As clinicians everywhere know, the management of each case is a team effort. It is no less true for texts like this one, and we have a number of people to thank for their assistance. First, we would like to express our sincere appreciation to our partners who put up with less support and time from us during the writing and editing of *Emergency Neurology*. There were also a number of colleagues at the University of California San Francisco (UCSF) who generously offered suggestions, answered questions, and supported this effort. We would like to express our gratitude to the UCSF Neurohospitalist Division faculty, who are each national leaders in the care of patients with complex and urgent neurological illnesses and are also exceptional teachers. UCSF is a very special medical institution, with seemingly an international expert in virtually every subject we wanted to be accurate about. We remain indebted to all of our colleagues here in the Neurology Department, and we could not think of more knowledgeable team to be part of. Any errors are ours, through misinterpretation or asking the wrong questions of them. Several editors at Oxford University Press helped on this project, including Jordan McAndrew and Craig Panner—many thanks to you all for being patient with us and alternately pushing us when that was needed. Finally, we would like to thank each other for the careful reading and editing of each other's chapters before we sent them in to Oxford University Press. Thanks Mo, thanks Sara!

Sara C. LaHue
Morris Levin

Emergency
Neurology

Diagnostic Dilemmas

1 Neurological Deficits Following Carotid Endarterectomy

A 68-year-old man who presented 6 days ago with transient language difficulty was found to have high-grade left internal carotid stenosis and then underwent left carotid endarterectomy (CAE) 3 days ago. Today he awoke with numbness in his right arm, which has persisted all morning. He also complains of a mild generalized headache. His wife called 911, and you are now seeing him the ER. Vital signs are normal, HEENT exams are normal, lungs are clear, and cardiac exam is normal. Neck is supple, and the endarterectomy incision is healing well. However, there is a bruit over this carotid. On neurological exam, his mental state, cranial nerves, strength, and coordination are all intact, but there does seem to be numbness over the entire right arm. CT scan without contrast is normal.

What do you do now?

Virtually every clinician treating adults knows that carotid endarterectomy (CEA) has been proven effective for treatment of symptomatic carotid stenosis. Fewer, however, have seen complications and feel comfortable dealing with them. It turns out that perioperative mortality can be as high as 3%, even at experienced centers. All of the usual potential postsurgical adverse consequences can occur in these patients. Wound dehiscence and infection are very rare. The most common adverse sequelae include myocardial infarction, transient ischemic attack (TIA)/stroke, hyperperfusion syndrome (HPS), neck region nerve injury, and parotitis. Stroke in the perioperative period can result from a number of contributing causes including platelet aggregation and thrombosis formation, plaque emboli, carotid dissection, and relatively low cerebral arterial perfusion pressure. The etiology of TIA or stroke must be assessed in order to choose the appropriate treatment.

After symptoms that could relate to carotid disease develop, the first step—and one which must be done quickly—is to rule out intracranial hemorrhage with head CT scan and then, if negative, to get a reliable visualization of the carotid artery over its cervical and intracranial course. This is best done via intraarterial angiography to detect flow-limiting dissection or thrombosis. CT angiography is often quicker and nearly as useful. If either is found, anti-coagulation had traditionally been the treatment of choice. High-quality duplex ultrasound evaluation can be helpful to confirm good flow through the proximal carotid and is used as a first step by some teams. Some surgeons favor surgical re-exploration if complications happen very early, with percutaneous carotid angioplasty with direct stenting. Many case reports document remission of neurological symptoms if stenting is done quickly, and several case series comparing stenting to surgical re-exploration attest to this.

Intraarterial thrombolytic therapy, in highly selected cases, may be another treatment option in patients with a postoperative thrombotic stroke suggested by arteriography. The rationale for the administration of tissue-type plasminogen activator (tPA) for these patients is based on its proven success in acute stroke, but there is no clear evidence to support its use here.

Myocardial infarction can occur after CEA, with incidence as high as 2%. Risk factors include older age, preexisting coronary artery disease, and peripheral arterial disease. Headaches are not uncommon after CEA and are often benign, but a severe headache should definitely prompt immediate medical attention. Contralateral stroke after CEA is rare but does occur, often for unclear reasons.

An important syndrome to exclude is HPS, which can produce three characteristic conditions: (1) persistent headache, (2) intracerebral hemorrhage, or (3) focal seizures. This last can involve significant post-seizure ("Todds") paralysis which can be misleading. HPS tends to occur 3–10 days following endarterectomy. The etiology of the HPS is thought to be caused by some degree of cerebral autoregulation breakdown due to the large change in flow. HPS seems to be more likely with high-grade (>80%) preoperative carotid occlusion and in patients with recent stroke. It might be difficult to differentiate hyperperfusion consequences from peri- or postoperative stroke. Head CT and MRI with T2 or FLAIR sequences typically show cerebral edema with or without intracerebral hemorrhage. Transcranial Doppler testing can reveal cerebral hyperperfusion in some cases. Strict control of systemic hypertension (systolic pressure <150 mmHg) is the best way to treat HPS and may require intravenous antihypertensives. Generally, the lability in postoperative blood pressure (BP) tends to resolve in the first 24 hours.

Since cranial nerves can be damaged during the operative procedure, this cause of neurological deficits must also be excluded if cranial nerve symptoms and signs tend to predominate (unlike the presenting case). Nerves at risk include (1) vagus nerve, which, if damaged, can lead to vocal cord paralysis; (2) portions of the facial nerve, leading to an asymmetric smile; (3) glossopharyngeal nerve which can lead to carotid sinus dysfunction, and, finally, (4) the hypoglossal nerve, which may result in dysarthria, and tongue deviation to the side of injury on examination. Nerve damage is generally due to traction, but intraoperative transection is also possible. The most reliable predictor of cranial nerve injury during endarterectomy is surgery duration, with a very low likelihood of cranial nerve damage in patients for whom OR time was less than 2 hours.

· CAE is generally safe but postoperative complications include stroke and hyperperfusion syndrome.

· In patients who develop focal deficits in the perioperative period, immediate CT of the head is recommended to exclude hemorrhage.

· Vascular imaging is essential to determine the presence of thrombosis or dissection of the carotid artery.

· Assessment of intracranial arterial blood flow is important in determining the presence of the hyperperfusion syndrome.

· Management of arterial BP is crucial if hyperperfusion syndrome is suspected.

Further Reading

Adhiyaman V, Alexander S. Cerebral hyperperfusion syndrome following carotid endarterectomy. *Q J Med.* 2007;100:239–244.

Anzuini A, Briguori C, Roubin G, Rosanio S, et al. Emergency stenting to treat neurological complications occurring after carotid endarterectomy. *J Am Coll Cardiol.* 2001;37:2074–2079.

Clouse WD, Ergul EA, Patel VI, Lancaster RT, LaMuraglia GM, Cambria RP, Conrad MF. Characterization of perioperative contralateral stroke after carotid endarterectomy. *J Vasc Surg.* 2017;66(5):1450–1456.

Farooq MU, Goshgarian C, Min J, Gorelick PB. Pathophysiology and management of reperfusion injury and hyperperfusion syndrome after carotid endarterectomy and carotid artery stenting. *Exp Translational Stroke Med.* 2016;8(1):7.

Flanigan DP, Flanigan ME, Dorne AL, et al. Long-term results of 442 consecutive, standardized carotid endarterectomy procedures in standard-risk and high-risk patients. *J Vasc Surg.* 2007;46:876.

Tu J, Wang S, Huo Z, Wu R, Yao C, Wang S. Repeated carotid endarterectomy versus carotid artery stenting for patients with carotid restenosis after carotid endarterectomy: Systematic review and meta-analysis. *Surgery.* 2015;57(6):1166–1173. doi:10.1016/j.surg.2015.02.005

2 Prolonged Migraine Aura

A 34-year-old woman, with a history of migraine attacks with aura, describes to the ER physician a typical migraine attack yesterday with scintillations and vision loss in the "left eye." She states that the headache abated with oral sumatriptan but the visual symptoms have not. The longest her migraine aura has lasted in the past is approximately 60 minutes. She feels anxious and a bit confused, but mental status testing is normal. Funduscopy is normal, and the ophthalmology consultant has excluded ocular disease. There does seem to be a left visual field deficit involving both upper and lower visual quadrants, but it tends to fluctuate. Cranial nerve exam is otherwise normal. Motor exam is normal. Sensory exam is generally normal, but there may be some diminution to light touch and vibration in the left arm and trunk. Coordination is intact; gait seems limited by vision. Routine labs are normal. CT of the head with and without contrast is normal.

What do you do now?

This patient has relatively typical migraine aura symptoms (visual and sensory) but of atypical duration. The *International Classification of Headache Disorders*, 3rd edition (International Headache Society [ICHD] 2018) defines prolonged migraine aura as lasting more than 1 week without radiographic evidence of infarction. A second entity, *migrainous stroke* is defined as "one or more aura symptoms [which] persisting for >60 minutes" and where "Neuroimaging demonstrates ischaemic infarction in a relevant area" (see Boxes 2.1 and 2.2). Thus, our patient fits neither definition. An important deciding diagnostic test is MRI with diffusion-weighted imaging (DWI). If this is positive, it is very possible that a migrainous stroke has occurred. Migraine itself is a mild risk factor for stroke, particularly in certain populations, most notably young women. This increased stroke risk is primarily limited to patients who experience migraine auras, although migraine without aura carries an overall mild increased risk of stroke as well. An unanswered question is whether a longer than average duration of aura symptoms magnifies the risk. Also unanswered, and of great interest, is the question of stroke pathophysiology in migraine. Presumably this is related either to some migraine-induced circulatory compromise or hypermetabolic "exhaustion" of normal perfusion, leading to relative ischemia to one or more brain regions.

But if the MRI is negative, there are still two important imperatives: (1) to continue to investigate possible causes of ischemia or other possible causes of prolonged aura-like symptoms and (2) to attempt to curtail

---

BOX 2.1   **International Classification of Headache Disorders, 3rd Edition: Persistent aura without infarction. Aura symptoms persisting for 1 week or more without evidence of infarction on neuroimaging**

Diagnostic criteria:

A. Aura fulfilling criterion B
B. Occurring in a patient with 1.2 *Migraine with aura* and typical of previous auras except that one or more aura symptoms persists for ≥1 week
C. Neuroimaging shows no evidence of infarction
D. Not better accounted for by another ICHD-3 diagnosis

> **BOX 2.2** **International Classification of Headache Disorders, 3rd Edition: Migrainous infarction. One or more migrainous aura symptoms associated with an ischemic brain lesion in appropriate territory demonstrated by neuroimaging**
>
> *Diagnostic criteria:*
>
> A. A migraine attack fulfilling criteria B and C
> B. Occurring in a patient with 1.2 *Migraine with aura* and typical of previous attacks except that one or more aura symptoms persists for >60 minutes
> C. Neuroimaging demonstrates ischemic infarction in a relevant area
> D. Not better accounted for by another ICHD-3 diagnosis

the aura. There are a number of conditions which may mimic prolonged auras including occipital lobe epilepsy, vertebrobasilar transient ischemic attacks, cerebral venous thrombosis, reversible cerebral vasoconstriction syndrome (RCVS), carotid or vertebral artery dissection, cerebral vasculitis, and hematological diseases causing "sludging." Mitochondrial encephalopathy, lactic acidosis, and stroke-like episodes syndrome (MELAS) and cerebral autosomal dominant arteriopathy with subcortical infarcts and leukoencephalopathy (CADASIL) are two other possibilities which MRI should exclude. CT angiography may be necessary in cases of prolonged aura to exclude vasculitis and RCVS. Imaging of the neck vessels with CT angiography (CTA) or MR angiography (MRA) may also be appropriate. EEG is very useful not only in excluding ongoing epileptic activity, but also to corroborate neurophysiological alterations in the cortex corresponding to the patient's symptoms. In the presenting patient, one would suspect to see some altered electrophysiological activity in right posterior derivations.

Persistent aura symptoms are rare but well-documented. They are often bilateral and may actually last for months or years. The 1-week minimum required by the ICHD is based on the opinion of experts, and solid evidence supporting this timing has not really be presented. Similarly, there are no clear treatment guidelines for patients suffering from prolonged migraine auras. Historically, despite a lack of evidence of real benefit, inhalation therapy with 10% carbon dioxide and 90% oxygen, amyl nitrate or isopro-terenol, and sublingual nifedipine have been used based on the theory that migrainous auras were the result of prolonged vasoconstriction. And recent studies of patients with prolonged migraine aura have found areas of cortical hypoperfusion corresponding to the region of aura symptoms. However, it seems that this is the result of a decreased metabolic demand rather than an ischemic mechanism, so presumably there is ongoing cortical spreading depression in these patients which might respond to a different therapeutic approach. Hence, a number of agents have been tried including magnesium sulfate, prochlorperazine, divalproex, acetazolamide, verapamil, flunarizine, lamotrigine, gabapentin, and memantine. Intravenous magnesium sulfate is probably a good place to start due to its relative safety, followed by intrave-nous divalproex. Selected patients with persistent aura have responded to occipital nerve blocks.

So, in summary, with prolonged migraine aura it is imperative to look further for evidence of cerebral ischemia and other causes of focal neu-rological deficits, which can then be explored and managed. If there is no stroke on MRI DWI images, prolonged aura is the best diagnosis. There are several options for treating the aura in hopes of curtailing it but no clear guidelines. Unfortunately, little is known currently about the etiology, risk factors, prognosis, and best treatments in prolonged migraine aura. Clearly, this presentation is concerning to patients, so migraine preventive strategies should be optimized.

KEY POINTS TO REMEMBER

- Migraine auras typically develop over 5–20 minutes and resolve within 1 hour or less.
- When aura lasts beyond 1 hour, investigation into other possible causes of focal neurological deficits should be considered.
- MRI with DWI should be abnormal in migrainous infarction, and MR or CT imaging along with EEG can generally rule out other pathological causes.

- Treatments which have helped some patients to halt prolonged auras include magnesium sulfate, divalproex, oxygen, and verapimil.

Further Reading

Cuadrado ML, Aledo-Serrano Á, López-Ruiz P, Gutiérrez-Viedma Á, Fernández C, Orviz A, Arias JA. Greater occipital nerve block for the acute treatment of prolonged or persistent migraine aura. *Cephalalgia.* 2017; 37(8):812–818.

Headache Classification Committee of the International Headache Society. International Classification of Headache Disorders, 3rd edition. *Cephalalgia.* 2018; 38:1–211.

Hu X, Zhou Y, Zhao H, Peng C. Migraine and the risk of stroke: an updated meta-analysis of prospective cohort studies. *Neurological Sciences.* 2017; 38(1):33–40.

Viana M, Sances G, Linde M, Nappi G, Khaliq F, Goadsby PJ, Tassorelli C. Prolonged migraine aura: new insights from a prospective diary-aided study. *J Headache pain.* 2018;19(1):77.

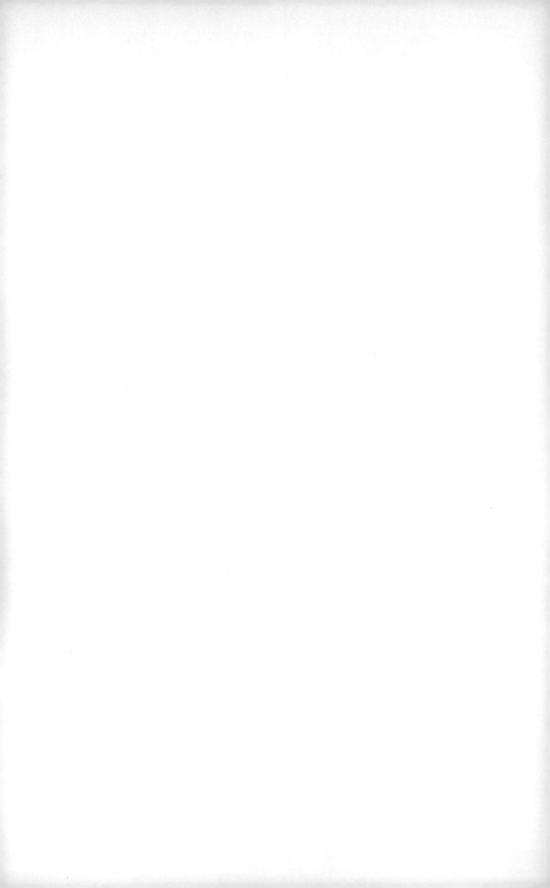

3 Acute Generalized Weakness

In the ED, a 28-year-old man complains of bilateral leg weakness for the past day and a half. He thinks it is due to a strenuous soccer match 2 days ago but feels that things seem to be worsening. He denies headache, visual problems, and any difficulty swallowing or breathing, but he also complains about some pain in his posterior thighs and back. He has had no bladder or bowel incontinence. He had a "cold" 2 weeks ago. He has been diagnosed with bipolar disorder and obsessive compulsive disorder and has been taking a combination of sodium divalproex and sertraline over the past 6 months. He also admits to frequent marijuana use and "some" alcohol use. An emergency medicine resident has examined this patient and found an entirely normal neurological exam. You repeat the exam and find that when asked to sit and stand, the patient has unexpected difficulty, and there is some impairment in gait. General exam is normal; there is no rash.

What do you do now?

While this case sounds like a standard presentation for Guillain-Barré syndrome (GBS, aka acute inflammatory demyelinating polyneuropathy), there are a few odd details. Against the diagnosis of GBS might be the normal reflexes, sparing of the upper extremities and face, and proximal location. On the other hand, GBS often begins with leg weakness, and, even though distal sensory complaints are the rule, many patients do complain of back pain. Reflexes, and upper body strength, may be normal for the first several days in GBS. Since the pathophysiology of GBS is thought to be an autoimmune attack on peripheral nerve myelin resulting from activation by an infectious agent (e.g., *Campylobacter*, *Mycoplasma*, and recently, Zika virus) with similar antigenic epitopes, a recent infection may be an important clue. Yet many patients with GBS cannot recall recent infections and conversely, the incidence of recent "colds" in the general population can be high.

Other possibilities for progressive weakness include myasthenia gravis, tick paralysis, Lyme neuropathy, HIV polyradiculoneuropathy, hypercalcemia, hypokalemia, hypothyroidism, heavy metal intoxication, drug toxicity, botulism, polymyositis, polio (highly unlikely in North America and Europe), and upper spinal cord lesions (see Box 3.1 for a more complete list).

Myasthenia rarely begins in the proximal lower extremities, and there is no history of instigators of a myasthenic syndrome in this patient. Botulism symptoms usually include blurred vision, nausea, abdominal pain (with ingestion), malaise, and/or dry mouth. Polymyositis should be apparent on lab testing (creatine kinase [CK], erythrocyte sedimentation rate [ESR], CBC). Electrolyte abnormalities can easily be ruled out, as can thyroid abnormalities and HIV infection. The patient was not taking medications known to cause generalized weakness. Lead neuropathy usually begins in the arms, and intoxication with arsenic and thallium usually causes GI symptoms as well. Porphyria can be ruled out with the absence of porphobilinogen on urinalysis. Lyme disease can indeed cause a polyradiculitis, and the pathognomonic bull's-eye rash may have been missed, but cranial nerve palsies are much more common. Also, CSF pleocytosis is seen. Tick paralysis is, however, a real possibility as he has been exposed to the common causes—wood ticks and dog ticks. The presentation is similar to GBS, but CSF protein concentration should be

Guillain-Barré syndrome
Myasthenia gravis
Myasthenia syndrome (e.g., aminoglycoside-induced)
Tick paralysis
Lyme neuropathy
HIV polyradiculoneuropathy
Hypercalcemia
Hypokalemia
Hypothyroidism
Heavy metal intoxication (arsenic, lead, thallium)
Medication (isoniazid [INH], vinca compounds, dapsone,
   nitrofurantoin)
Botulism
Sarcoidosis
Polymyositis
Polio
Porphyria
Spinal cord lesions

normal. Tick paralysis is caused by a toxin that seems to interfere with ace-tylcholine release at the neuromuscular junction and abates soon after the tick is removed. Therefore, a search for ticks is recommended, including the hair.

A common question is how far to proceed in searching for a spinal cord lesion in a patient like this one. After all, he did play a highly physical sport the day symptoms began. The lack of reflex change and bowel/bladder dysfunction argues against this etiology, but it is difficult to be sure in these cases. Given the absence of arm weakness, at minimum a thoracic spine MRI should be obtained, though some may argue for a complete spinal MRI. A key test in this case is lumbar puncture to see if CSF protein is high. Unfortunately, in the first week of GBS, around one-third of patients have normal CSF. Neurophysiological testing is also helpful, though usually more fruitful within a week or two of symptom onset, specifically showing slowed motor conduction along with absent F and H waves. Serologic testing for anti-ganglioside antibodies associated with GBS and its variants should be considered.

So, despite a high clinical suspicion for the diagnosis of GBS, a number of mimics exist, and workup needs to be thorough. Admission to the hospital for further investigation, treatment, and monitoring is generally most efficient and safe. Respiratory power should be monitored frequently with forced vital capacity (FVC) and mean inspiratory force (MIF), with a low threshold to consider elective intubation. If testing is confirmatory of GBS, IVIg administration is generally begun unless symptoms are extremely mild. Plasma exchange is an alternative but since it is more difficult and less available, IVIg has largely replaced it for the treatment of GBS in many institutions. Prognosis is generally very good for recovery, although the majority of patients will have some residual motor deficits.

KEY POINTS TO REMEMBER

- Acute Guillain-Barré syndrome may present in atypical fashion, without clear history of antecedent infection.
- The differential diagnosis in acute diffuse weakness is large, with a number of entities producing similar symptomatology.
- A good initial workup should include thorough metabolic screening as well as CSF analysis.
- Spinal imaging should be done early if there is any suspicion of myelopathy.

Further Reading

Fahoum F, Drory V, Issakov J, Neufeld MY. Neurosarcoidosis presenting as Guillain-Barre-like syndrome: a case report and review of the literature. *J Clin Neuromusc Dis.* 2009;11:35–43.

Krishnan AV, Lin CS, Reddel SW, Mcgrath R, Kiernan MC. Conduction block and impaired axonal function in tick paralysis. *Muscle & Nerve.* 2009;40:358–362.

Wijdicks EF, Klein CJ. Guillain-Barre syndrome. *Mayo Clinic Proc.* 2017;92:467–479.

4   Syncope

A 78-year-old woman had an episode of loss of consciousness at home yesterday afternoon. She admitted this to her daughter this morning when asked about the cut on her head. She later admitted to several ("maybe half a dozen?") previous episodes of loss of consciousness, some of which led to falls, over the past 3–4 years. She feels fine now, although she is anxious. She denies incontinence of urine or feces. She did experience a mild headache when recovering from her syncopal attack yesterday, but "it's gone now." Her medical history includes mild COPD and controlled hypertension. Her blood pressure now is 148/78, does not drop significantly on sitting or standing, and her pulse is 88 and regular. Respirations are 14 per minute, and she is afebrile. Neurological exam is intact including mental status, cranial nerves, strength, reflexes, coordination, and gait. She asks you why this happened and worries about the possibility of it happening again, "maybe even when I am driving!"

What do you do now?

The conscious patient reporting syncope is one of the most frequent triggers for both neurological and cardiological consultation in the ED. The first step is to determine if, in fact, this was actual syncope (brief loss of consciousness). Some patients will ultimately be found to have had transient loss of vision, lightheadedness (presyncope), or transient confusion. If there was a transient loss of consciousness, and this can be corroborated by witnesses or perhaps by evidence of trauma sustained due a fall which often accompanies syncope, the next step is to attempt to discover clues to the cause of the loss of consciousness. Box 4.1 lists causes of loss of consciousness which include those due to reduced cardiac output.

BOX 4.1   **Causes of brief loss of consciousness**

Cardiac arrhythmia
Myocardial infarction
Pericarditis or cardiac tamponade
Cardiomyopathy
Aortic stenosis
Mitral valve stenosis or prolapse or atrial myxoma
Dissecting aortic aneurysm
Orthostatic hypotension
Carotid sinus syncope
Vasovagal syncope
Pneumothorax
Pulmonary stenosis
Pulmonary hypertension
Pulmonary embolus
Basilar artery occlusion
Stroke
Subclavian steal syndrome
Intracerebral or subarachnoid hemorrhage
Hypoglycemia
Anemia
Hypoxemia
Hypercarbia
Psychogenic

Important historical features to obtain include information about provocative factors: after standing, after exercise, while overheated, in the bathroom, after eating, with stress or intense emotion, or following neck position changes. Associated symptoms to list include changes in thinking, nausea, palpitations, shortness of breath, chest pain, and incontinence. A thorough list of medications should be obtained, and a urine toxicology screen is not a bad idea. Electrocardiography is essential, and a plain CT scan of the head is generally necessary, particularly if there is any suspicion of head injury.

In the presenting case stroke is unlikely as neurological exam is normal, and hemorrhage has been ruled out by a negative CT of the head. Posterior cerebral circulation occlusive disease is possible but is unlikely in the absence of typical accompanying symptoms such as vertigo, imbalance, dysarthria, facial numbness, and visual loss. MRI of the brain as well as vascular imaging (either MR or CT angiography) can help to exclude this.

Intermittent arrhythmias which reduce cardiac output can be occult but cardiac rhythm monitoring, via inpatient telemetry or portable monitoring systems, generally clarifies the presence of this as a cause. Blood pressure (BP) should be checked in both arms to investigate the possibility of subclavian stenosis/coarctation leading perhaps to subclavian steal. A strong clue to this pathophysiology is instigation of syncopal sensations by exercising the ipsilateral arm, promoting "stealing" of blood from the brain via the vertebral artery to supply the arm. Chest x-ray and echocardiography will help to rule out pericarditis, tamponade, mitral valve, aortic valve or atrial pathology, and cardiomyopathy. Hypotension, venous engorgement, weak pulse, and findings on cardiac auscultation might also be present with cardiac disease.

Orthostatic hypotension (OH) should be relatively straightforward to rule out. A drop in diastolic pressure of more than 10 mm Hg, or systolic of 20 mm Hg, when the patient sits or stands up, is diagnostic. If orthostatic tachycardia occurs, one suspects hypovolemia; if not, there may be an element of dysautonomia. The potential causes of OH include drug effects (anticholinergics, dopaminergics, and diuretics), autonomic neuropathies (e.g., diabetes or amyloid neuropathy), Parkinson's disease and "Parkinson-plus" syndromes (including multisystem atrophy), hypovolemia, and anemia. If OH is identified, these possibilities should all be investigated.

Vasovagal syncope, also referred to as *neurocardiogenic syncope*, is caused by a relative surge in parasympathetic activity precipitated by emotional stress, fear, excessive coughing, pain, or, in some cases, urination (micturition syncope). Bradycardia and hypotension lead to brain hypoperfusion. Premonitory symptoms can include diaphoresis, pallor, and nausea. This may be the most common cause of syncope and is essentially a diagnosis of exclusion until the patient notices a pattern of recurrence in similar situations. When vasovagal syncope results from autonomic hypersensitivity to position changes, it begins to resemble orthostatic hypotension. Using a tilt table to incline the patient during monitoring for BP and pulse rate can be diagnostic. Treatment includes avoidance of triggers, volume expansion tactics, and medications.

Chest or abdominal pain and/or dyspnea should be present to at least some degree in myocardial infarction, pneumothorax, dissecting aortic aneurysm, and pulmonary embolism. Measuring levels of cardiac enzymes should be considered. Anemia, hypoxemia, hypercarbia, and other metabolic disturbances can be easily ruled out with routine labs and pulse oximetry. Carotid sinus syncope occurs when the carotid sinus is compressed by a tight collar, a seat belt, backpack strap, or other source of external pressure. This results in vagal stimulation leading to bradycardia and vasodilation with resulting systemic hypotension.

Seizures, when generalized, usually cause loss of consciousness or at least a period of unresponsiveness to one's environment. A key to the diagnosis here is postictal alteration in mentation, consciousness, or other neurological function. Patients tend to recover pretty quickly after cardiovascular syncope, but much less so following generalized seizures. Other important clues are witnesses' reports of sustained motor movements, evidence of tongue biting, and incontinence. Interestingly, causes of syncope which involve some degree of cerebral hypoxia can cause tonic-clonic movements briefly, mimicking epileptic seizures.

Drug intoxication is always a possibility although a classic syncopal event is unlikely. Still, drug screening must be considered. Psychogenic syncope is seen in patients with depression, anxiety, and panic. Vasovagal mechanisms, hyperventilation, or somatization may be the proximate cause in these patients.

So, there are a number of possibilities here, including several relatively unlikely neurological ones. The neurologist who can reason through these cases and offer advice other than "order an EEG" will be much respected and appreciated.

KEY POINTS TO REMEMBER

- Syncope can result from many causes including cardiovascular, pulmonary, metabolic, neurological, and psychogenic.
- Careful general, cardiac, pulmonary, neurological history and exams are essential, including careful assessment of pulse and BP bilaterally and in different positions.
- Laboratory investigation should include metabolic and hematological panels, and cardiac enzymes. ECG, chest x-ray, EEG, echocardiography, and cardiac monitoring should be part of the investigation as well as CT of the head, particularly if there is any suspicion of head injury.
- Cerebrovascular imaging of the head and neck should likewise be considered in cases of syncope accompanied by any focal neurological deficits.

Further Reading

Chen-Scarabelli C, Scarabelli TM. Neurocardiogenic syncope. *BMJ*. 2004;329:336–341.

Moya A, Sutton R, Ammirati F, et al. Guidelines for the diagnosis and management of syncope. *Eur Heart J*. 2009;30:2631–2671.

Serrano LA, Hess EP, Bellolio MF, et al. Accuracy and quality of clinical decision rules for syncope in the emergency department: a systematic review and meta-analysis. *Ann Emerg Med*. 2010;56:362–373.

5   Monocular Visual Loss

A 46-year-old laboratory tech is seen for acute
visual loss in the right eye. She states that vision
seemed normal yesterday, and she did not even
notice it today until she tried closing her left eye.
She has had no recent infection or trauma. She
is on no daily medication. She denies pain in the
eye and headache. General exam is normal: vital
signs are normal; neck is supple; lungs, heart
and abdomen are normal; there is no skin rash.
Ocular exam is normal, without papilledema,
but pupillary reactivity to light on the right
shows a relative afferent pupillary defect (RAPD).
Neurological exam otherwise normal. Routine
labs are normal.

What do you do now?

Acute vision loss is a daunting presentation. Rapid identification of the cause and speedy corrective measures are imperative. Fortunately for neurologists, the answers are usually clarified by ophthalmologists, but a common reason for consultation arises when "ocular causes have been ruled out."

The differential diagnosis of acute monocular vision loss can be divided into the following categories (beginning with the most peripheral and moving more centrally): (1) opacities in the cornea, lens, or vitreous humor; (2) retinal disease; (3) retinal or eye ischemia; (4) optic nerve disease (ischemic, compressive, or demyelinating); (5) pathology of the chiasm; and (6) conversion, factitious disorder, or malingering.

Ocular opacities like corneal edema or vitreous hemorrhage generally do not cause a Marcus Gunn pupil (relative afferent pupillary defect—RAPD) even with dramatic visual blurring or loss. They are generally painless. Funduscopic exam is generally diagnostic when done by an ophthalmologist. Iritis and uveitis can obscure vision due to localized edema, but eye pain and obvious ocular inflammation generally lead these patients to where they need to be: into the hands of an ophthalmologist. Acute retinal detachment is usually painless and begins with some degree of vitreous detachment with patients complaining of "floaters." Retinal detachment may eventually cause a deafferented pupil, but generally not initially. Complaints usually begin with peripheral field loss. Regular funduscopic exam is often negative although occasionally one can see the classic white "billowing" retinal separation. A dilated eye exam by an ophthalmologist is usually diagnostic.

Ischemia of the retina can arise in the setting of several different disease states. Amaurosis fugax (transient loss of vision in one eye) occurs usually in the form of a "shade coming down" then receding. This generally arises as the result of atherosclerotic or thrombotic emboli to the central retinal artery or one of its retinal branches from a diseased carotid artery. Occasionally one can see small atheromatous or calcific fragments in retinal arteries on funduscopic exam. If the embolus becomes lodged long enough, retinal ischemic injury can occur, leading to permanent visual impairment. Retinal artery occlusion may cause deafferentation. Funduscopic exam usually reveals an area of pallor on the retina with a red macula due to its thinner epithelium. There is little or no effective treatment for this condition although hydration, assurance of optimal carotid system perfusion, and perhaps ocular massage may help. Searching for the specific etiology and treatment of it is of course imperative in hopes of preventing further brain ischemia. More proximal embolic or atheromatous occlusion of the ophthalmic artery may also cause monocular vision loss and can, like strokes elsewhere, occur on the basis of cardiac, paradoxical, or arterial embolization; arterial thrombosis; or atherosclerotic narrowing.

Central retinal vein occlusion (RVO) is another fairly frequent cause of acute monocular vision loss and is generally diagnosed funduscopically by seeing multiple retinal hemorrhages and papilledema. The vision loss is often not as severe as that resulting from arterial occlusion. Despite many proposed interventions, there are no treatments proven to reopen occluded retinal veins. Management is directed at secondary complications of RVO that affect vision, including macular edema, retinal neovascularization, and anterior segment neovascularization. Temporal arteritis (TA; giant cell arteritis) affects the temporal artery and extradural portions of the carotid and vertebral arteries. This includes the ophthalmic artery so visual loss can occur as a result of resulting ischemia to the retina and/or optic nerve. TA usually presents with severe headache and often polymyalgia rheumatica (manifested by diffuse aching, muscle stiffness, and flu-like symptoms), and occasionally one can detect a tender temporal artery. By the time vision has been impaired, it is probably too late to save what has been lost but rapid treatment with intravenous steroids can prevent further loss. Retinal vasculitis can also produce monocular visual impairment and is diagnosed with dilated funduscopic exam and flourescein angiography. The condition is usually painless. Etiology is often not discovered, but management consists of searching for systemic causes of vasculitis and treatment with immunosuppressants.

Anterior ischemic optic neuropathy (AION) is due to ischemia and generally occurs in patients with diabetes, hypertension, or lupus. Papilledema is often seen. Treatment is aimed at the underlying disease(s), and patients often improve. Alternatively, the rarer posterior ischemic optic neuropathy (PION) does not produce papilledema. It may be due to vasculitis, as can AION, and the diagnosis is usually made by exclusion of other causes. Both AION and PION can be caused by TA.

Optic neuritis (ON) due to acute demyelination is often painful and usually causes a deafferentated pupil early, along with the vision loss. Papilledema is seen when the inflammation is close to the retina, but when it is retrobulbar, diagnosis rests on clinical suspicion along with brain MRI findings, and enhanced MRI can reveal optic nerve inflammation. Standard treatment is methylprednisolone. ON can be seen as an isolated syndrome (although there is a significant chance of developing MS), as an exacerbation of MS, or as the presentation of one of the neuromyelitis optica spectrum disorders (NMOSD) as opposed to just NMO, which includes autoimmune diseases with antibodies to aquaporin-4 (AQP4) and myelin oligodendrocyte glycoprotein (MOG). Leber optic neuropathy is inherited mitochondrially and can lead to unilateral optic neuropathy either subacutely or acutely. Subsequent involvement of the other eye is the rule. There is no treatment known.

Mass lesions or infections affecting the optic nerve in the orbit or in the region of the optic foramen generally progress more slowly with gradual visual impairment over weeks or longer. Involvement of the optic chiasm by neoplastic and infectious diseases does not lead to monocular vision loss but rather bitemporal or homonymous field deficits.

Conversion disorder may cause monocular blindness, but it is more often binocular and can be detected fairly easily by normal pupillary reactivity, normal optokinetic strip testing, and normal visual evoked potentials. Similarly, visual loss due to malingering or factitious disorder is suggested by these findings on examination. Clinical suspicion arises when secondary gain is present.

Diagnostic workup, once thorough ophthalmological examination has been done and found to be normal, should include complete blood count, erythrocyte sedimentation rate (ESR), C-reactive protein, antinuclear antibody, hemoglobin A1C, brain MRI with contrast, dedicated carotid imaging, and echocardiogram. If suspicion for demyelinating disease is high, NMO, AQP4, and MOG antibodies should be checked. If the diagnosis is not clear, Lyme titer, HIV screen, lumbar puncture with CSF exam to include protein, glucose, fungal and TB stains, and cultures, oligoclonal, bands and IgG index should be done.

- Ophthalmological evaluation is critical in acute monocular visual loss and should include a dilated funduscopic exam (*prior to which* careful pupillary testing should be done).
- When ophthalmological causes of monocular blindness have been excluded, retinal ischemia, ischemic optic neuritis, and demyelinating optic neuritis must be considered.
- Diagnostic testing should include brain and vascular imaging, ESR, and possibly lumbar puncture.

Further Reading

Abbatemarco JR, Patell R, Buccola J, Willis MA. Acute monocular vision loss: don't lose sight of the differential. *Clev Clin J Med*. 2017;84(10):779.

Vortmann M, Schneider JI. Acute monocular visual loss. *Emerg Med Clin N Am*. 2008;26:73–96.

Ward TN, Levin M. Headache in giant cell arteritis and other arteritides. *Neurol Sci*. 2005;26(Suppl 2):s134–s137.

Zhang LY, Zhang J, Kim RK, et al. Risk of acute ischemic stroke in patients with monocular vision loss of vascular etiology. *J Neuro-Ophthal*. 2018;38(3):328–333.

6 Thunderclap Headache

A 42-year-old man rapidly developed a severe headache while biking up a challenging hill. He had to get off his bike, and then he called 911, which led to his arrival in the ED by ambulance. He told the ED staff that he has never had headaches and that this one "made me see stars." Pain continues for the next 2 hours along with some blurred vision. General and neurological exams are normal. Neck is supple and funduscopic exam is normal. CT of the head and lumbar puncture (LP) have been done and are negative.

What do you do now?

This is, of course, the famous "thunderclap headache." Most patients will seek attention, and some will turn out to have one of the scarier conditions that are known to cause sudden severe headaches, such as intracerebral hemorrhage or subarachnoid hemorrhage, which are identified with CT and LP (see Box 6.1). Seeing "stars" and complaining of persistent visual difficulties are clues that there may indeed be an underlying secondary cause of headache here. So—what is a wise course of action when this initial workup is negative? One problem is that several causes of thunderclap headache are identifiable only with more advanced imaging. Cerebral venous thrombosis is one example, since standard MRI imaging may fail to identify even large thrombi in cerebral veins. MR or CT venography, however is almost always diagnostic. The syndrome of reversible cerebral vasoconstriction syndrome (RCVS), also known as *Call-Fleming syndrome,* often presents as sudden or severe headache and only later with neurological deficits. Unlike CNS vasculitis, CSF in RCVS is generally normal, and

---

BOX 6.1   Causes of sudden (thunderclap) headache

- Acute hypertension
- Carotid or vertebral artery dissection
- Cerebral vasculitis
- Cerebral venous thrombosis
- Hypertensive, lobar, or pituitary intracranial hemorrhage
- Intracranial hypotension
- Primary thunderclap headache
- Reversible cerebral vasoconstriction syndrome (RCVS)
- Sphenoid sinusitis
- Subarachnoid hemorrhage or "aneurysmal leak" (sentinel headache)

Rarer causes

- Aqueductal stenosis
- Cardiac cephalalgia
- Colloid cyst of the third ventricle
- Giant cell arteritis
- Ischemic stroke

MRI is often normal as well. The hallmark is the finding of segmental arterial narrowing seen on angiography. Fortunately, CT angiography seems to be almost as useful as standard intraarterial angiography. Interestingly, RCVS often becomes symptomatic (with severe headache) after vigorous exercise and this may well be the explanation for this patient's presentation. To complicate matters, RCVS may lead to focal subarachnoid bleeding (perhaps the most common cause of acute severe headaches in these patients), which can lead to a fruitless quest for a ruptured aneurysm. While in most cases RCVS is a self-limited disorder, it may progress, and calcium channel blockers are often used in some centers to prevent stroke.

Carotid or vertebral arterial dissection can present with acute severe headache, without other neurological symptoms. Again, vascular imaging, including the proximal segments of these vessels, is required for exclusion of dissection. Sphenoid sinusitis may also present as sudden diffuse head pain, and, while it may be missed on CT, MRI is generally quite adequate to diagnose it. Spontaneous intracranial hypotension, generally diagnosed by the patient's complaint of significant worsening of pain upon sitting or standing and improvement with reclining, may present with thunderclap headache. Exertional headaches are generally short-lived, but exercise-induced migraine may persist, similar to regular migraine, for hours to even days. Likewise, orgasmic headache, thought to represent a benign primary headache type, can persist and mimic serious vascular causes. A key distinguishing feature, of course, is that these follow a pattern—stereotypic recurring sudden or at least rapidly building global headaches at or near the time of orgasm—clearly not the cause in our case. And finally, there is a primary benign headache condition termed "primary thunderclap headache," which is obviously a diagnosis of exclusion. Rare causes are possible, including third ventricular colloid cysts, giant cell arteritis, pheochromocytoma, and cardiac cephalgia due to an as yet unclear pain referral phenomenon from ischemic myocardium.

But have we really excluded an aneurysm as an underlying cause of this patient's severe acute headache? Head CT imaging resolution is generally considered adequate to detect subarachnoid blood (Figure 6.1). But some reports suggest that there are between 1% and 5% false negatives. Hence, the need for LP. But this, too, has a finite false-positive rate, particularly if the hemorrhage was recent, deep, and limited. There have been several

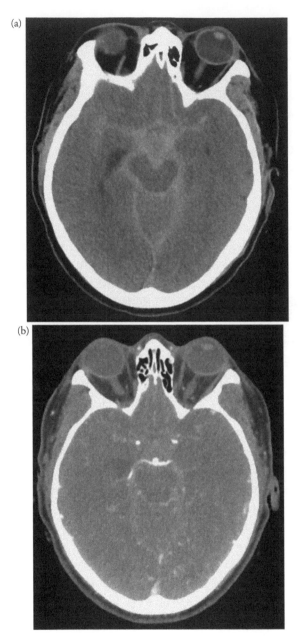

FIGURE 6.1 CT scan of a patient with subarachnoid hemorrhage (a) Axial view without contrast showing the presence of blood in the cerebral subarachnoid systems and (b) Axial view after contrast showing a basilar tip aneurysm.

reports of patients with *unruptured* aneurysms, or aneurysms which have "leaked," and produced thunderclap headaches (the so-called sentinel headache) without producing bloody CSF. MRI is generally very sensitive to even small amounts of subarachnoid blood, undetectable by CT or in the CSF sample. But high-resolution cerebrovascular imaging is necessary to exclude the possibility of an unruptured aneurysm. The mechanism underlying acute headache with unruptured aneurysm is not clear, but some have postulated stretching of the nociceptive receptors in the aneurysmal wall as causal. The International Classification of Headache Disorders also included unruptured arteriovenous malformation as a cause of headache, but these are generally not thunderclap in presentation.

So, what is the most parsimonious workup for thunderclap headache once CT and LP have been negative? A brain MRI to rule out recent hemorrhage, MRA of the cerebral vessels to investigate for aneurysm (or AVM) and segmental arterial narrowing, MRA of the cervical vessels to look for dissection and an MR venogram to rule out CVT would be a very thorough approach. MR angiography may not be as sensitive as CT angiography for detecting berry aneurysms, so the latter or a conventional intraarterial dye angiogram should be considered.

If all serious causes of thunderclap headache are ruled out, primary thunderclap headache may be the diagnosis although it must be viewed with suspicion. Indomethacin may relieve this type of headache, but opioids may be necessary.

KEY POINTS TO REMEMBER

- Sudden severe headache is a potential emergency and should be evaluated with CT and, if negative, LP to rule out hemorrhage.
- There are several diagnostic possibilities for thunderclap headache that may not be diagnosed with CT, LP, or even MRI, including cerebral arteritis, cerebral venous thrombosis, RCVS and cervical arterial dissection.
- Primary thunderclap headache, thought to be a primary headache disorder, may be the underlying diagnosis but must be a diagnosis of exclusion.

Further Reading

Barritt A, Miller S, Davagnanam I, Matharu M. Rapid diagnosis vital in thunderclap headache. *Practitioner.* 2016;260(1792):23–28.

Day JW, Raskin NH. Thunderclap headache: symptom of unruptured cerebral aneurysm. *Lancet* 1986;2(8518):1247–1248.

Ducros A, Wolff V. The typical thunderclap headache of reversible cerebral vasoconstriction syndrome and its various triggers. *Headache.* 2016;56(4):657–673.

Kowalski RG, Claassen J, Kreiter KT, et al. Initial misdiagnosis and outcome after subarachnoid hemorrhage. *JAMA.* 2004;291:866–869.

Singhal AB. Diagnostic challenges in RCVS, PACNS, and other cerebral arteriopathies. *Cephalalgia.* 2011;31:1067–1070.

7 Generalized Convulsive Status Epilepticus

A 45-year-old woman with a history of traumatic brain injury and alcohol use disorder was brought to an outside hospital by paramedics after having a witnessed seizure in the supermarket. She had a second seizure that was described as "generalized" en route to the hospital, and so she received midazolam 10 mg IM. She had a third generalized seizure in the outside hospital ED, and so she was intubated and loaded with fosphenytoin IV. Her vital signs were notable for a temperature of 100.2°F, blood pressure of 85/50, heart rate of 110, oxygenating well. Her exam was limited as she received paralytics in order to be intubated, but her pupils were reactive and symmetric to light; she was not following commands prior to intubation. Given concern for meningoencephalitis she was started on meningeal-dosed antibiotics. She underwent a head CT that showed a subdural hemorrhage; vessel imaging was unremarkable. She is transferred to your hospital for continuous EEG monitoring.

What do you do now?

Generalized convulsive status epilepticus (GCSE) is a neurological emergency with high morbidity and mortality. While the duration of seizure activity that defines GCSE has changed over time, it is clear that the sooner the seizure activity is stopped, the better the prognosis. The hippocampus is particularly sensitive to prolonged generalized seizure activity. For this reason, it is more practical to recommend prompt treatment for seizure activity lasting for at least 5 minutes, or two or more sequential seizures without full recovery of consciousness between seizures.

General support must include close scrutiny of airway, breathing, and circulation and monitoring of temperature as many patients in GCSE can become hyperthermic, leading to secondary brain injury (see Box 7.1). Acidosis usually occurs but resolves with termination of the seizure. Cardiac arrhythmias can also occur.

The most common cause of GCSE is discontinuation of medications, but new exacerbating factors must always be ruled out. Therefore, it is important to search for infection, including meningitis or encephalitis; metabolic derangements including aberrancies in levels of sodium (low), glucose (high/low), calcium (low), and magnesium (low); hepatic and renal

---

BOX 7.1 **An approach to status epilepticus**

1. Assess airway, breathing, and circulation
   Obtain finger-stick glucose: if glucose < 60 mg/dL then give thiamine 200 mg IV followed by D50W IV.
   Start IV with normal saline and obtain labs (CBC, BMP, Mg/Ca, LFTs, AED levels, ABG, toxicology screen).
2. Lorazepam 4 mg IV (2 mg/min) or midazolam 5–10 mg IM.
   Repeat benzodiazepine after 5–10 minutes if needed.
3. Give one of the following:
   • Fosphenytoin (20 mgPE/kg, maximum 1,500 mgPE)
   • Valproate (40 mg/kg, maximum 3,000 mg)
   • Levetiracetam (60 mg/kg, maximum 4,500 mg)
   Begin EEG monitoring if patient does not awaken or if anticipate escalation to continuous IV therapy.
4. Intubate and proceed to use of anesthetics.

dysfunction; drug toxicity (e.g., cocaine, amphetamines); ethanol or barbiturate withdrawal; hypoxia; and focal intracranial processes like ischemic or hemorrhagic stroke; subarachnoid or subdural hemorrhage (as seen in this case, see Figure 7.1); traumatic brain injury; or mass lesion. Convulsive movements can be observed in patients with basilar artery occlusions and so vigilance for this mimic is crucial.

Initial workup is done simultaneously with administration of antiepileptic drugs (AEDs) and should generally include an ABG, comprehensive metabolic panel, complete blood count, drug screen, urinalysis, and CT of the head. A lumbar puncture should be considered if this is a first seizure, first episode of GCSE, there is evidence of fever, or suspicion for subarachnoid hemorrhage. Complications from prolonged convulsive seizure should also be assessed, such as aspiration using chest x-ray, and rhabdomyolysis using serum creatine kinase.

In addition to providing rapid treatment, it will be important to make sure the patient is medically stable, and to ensure airway patency.

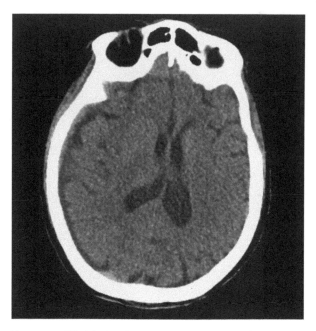

FIGURE 7.1 Noncontrast CT of the head showing acute-on-chronic right holohemispheric subdural hematoma with leftward midline shift.

Lorazepam 4 mg IV or midazolam IM (5 mg for patients 13–40 kg, and 10 mg for patients >40 kg) can be given acutely. There are now three AEDs shown to have similar efficacy for status epilepticus based on results from the Established Status Epilepticus Treatment Trial (ESETT). These AEDs are fosphenytoin (20 mgPE/kg, maximum 1,500 mgPE), valproate (40 mg/kg, maximum 3,000 mg), or levetiracetam (60 mg/kg, maximum 4,500 mg). The appropriate dose of these medications can be remembered by the 20-40-60 rule. The recommended loading dose of levetiracetam for GCSE is quite high, and so an alternate AED should be considered if the patient has renal impairment. If available, fosphenytoin is preferred to phenytoin as it can be administered faster and does not carry the risk of "purple-glove syndrome."

A finger stick glucose should be obtained quickly, and if glucose is lower than 60 mg/dL give thiamine 200 mg IV followed by D50W IV. If the patient is on INH or hydralazine, administer pyridoxine (vitamin B6) 5 g IV over 5 minutes, then repeat 30 minutes later.

If seizures continue, intubation should be considered given the likely need to escalate to anesthetics. It is reasonable to escalate to an anesthetic rather than additional trials of second-line AEDs. Advocate for short-acting paralytics if intubation is necessary to limit its impact on the neurological

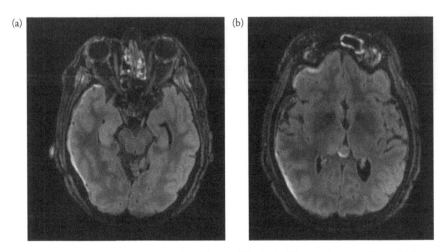

FIGURE 7.2 MRI of the brain showing signal abnormalities in the bilateral hippocampi (a) and right thalamus (b) likely due to postictal state.

exam. If available, EEG monitoring should be sought if seizure activity returns when sedatives are paused, or if there is a need to escalate continuous IV therapy. If EEG monitoring is not available, transfer to a facility that can provide continuous EEG monitoring should be attempted. MRI can also be helpful with identifying an underlying cause, and may also reveal post-ictal changes (Figure 7.2).

KEY POINTS TO REMEMBER

- Prompt treatment for GCSE is necessary for any seizure lasting at least 5 minutes or when there is an incomplete return to baseline between seizures.
- Control of seizures must be achieved as quickly as possible, along with a search for causes including meningitis, stroke/ hemorrhage, drug intoxication/withdrawal, metabolic derangements or head trauma.
- It is important to not underdose benzodiazepines if someone is in GCSE.
- There is a choice of three AEDs to load for GCSE: fosphenytoin (20 mgPE/kg, maximum 1,500 mgPE), valproate (40 mg/kg, maximum 3,000 mg), or levetiracetam (60 mg/kg, maximum 4,500 mg).
- General medical monitoring for hyperthermia, hypertension, hypoxia, renal dysfunction, electrolyte imbalance, and arrhythmia must occur simultaneously with treatment of GCSE.

Further Reading

Betjemann JP, Lowenstein DH. Status epilepticus in adults. *Lancet Neurol.* Jun 2015;14(6):615–624.

Kapur J, Elm J, Chamberlain JM, et al. Randomized trial of three anticonvulsant medications for status epilepticus. *N Engl J Med.* 2019;381(22):2103–2113. doi:10.1056/NEJMoa1905795

Silbergleit R, Durkalski V, Lowenstein D, et al. Intramuscular versus intravenous therapy for prehospital status epilepticus. *N Engl J Med.* 2012;366(7):591–600. doi:10.1056/NEJMoa1107494

Hospital-Acquired Delirium

A 72-year-old man with a history of a left frontal glioblastoma multiforme (GBM) had a witnessed generalized seizure shortly after dinner. He received midazolam by the paramedics and stopped seizing. On arrival to the ED, his blood pressure (BP) was 141/75, heart rate 105 and regular, and he was afebrile. His general examination revealed a laceration on the lateral aspect of his tongue. His neurological exam showed intact orientation but impaired naming and bilateral hearing impairment, as well as mild right face and hand weakness. A head CT showed increased edema around the GBM without hemorrhage. He received a levetiracetam load and dexamethasone. He was admitted to the hospital and stayed awake much of the night. He pulled at his IV, so limb restraints were placed. On hospital day 2, he said the year was "1953." That evening, he asked his wife to take their dog out for a bathroom break and gestured to the corner.

What do you do now?

There are many reasons why someone may become confused in the hospital. While confusion may seem innocuous, serious illness may underlie it. It is important to start with an assessment of the patient's airway, breathing, and circulation. Check vital signs, looking for abnormalities in BP and pulse (elevated or depressed), oxygen saturation, and temperature. Vital signs may point toward dehydration, hypertensive emergency, hypoxemia, or infection. A finger-stick glucose can be helpful to rule out hypoglycemia. If the patient is hypoglycemic, give thiamine prior to dextrose to avoid possible precipitation of Wernicke's encephalopathy. Review hospital medications, paying particular attention to anticholinergic medications, benzodiazepines, opioids, cefepime or other antibiotics, and steroids. If the patient is somnolent and there is recent opiate use, consider a naloxone trial (1–2 amps IV or IM every 5 minutes). If altered mental status develops within a few days of admission, compare inpatient medications with home medications to check for possible withdrawal, especially if the patient previously took benzodiazepines, opioids, or baclofen.

The bedside general physical examination should focus on screening for infectious signs, such as heart murmur, respiratory difficulty, and skin lesions/rashes. Meningismus should be looked for, though development of a new central nervous system infection during hospitalization is rare unless the altered mental status was present on admission or the patient has had neurosurgery or is immunocompromised.

The neurological exam can also help narrow the differential. The exam should include detailed mental status testing, especially attention (such as digit span forward and backward). Testing of language fluency, naming, repetition, and comprehension may point toward a receptive aphasia caused by a vascular or structural cause, which can be easily mistaken for "confusion" if the deficit is isolated to language without obvious motor deficits. The development of neglect is also a reason for altered mental status and should be checked. Pupil abnormalities can suggest a structural or toxic etiology. Cranial nerve dysfunction can suggest brainstem involvement or a process in the subarachnoid space. In addition to strength testing, which can indicate a hemispheric abnormality, it can also be helpful to assess for abnormal tone, involuntary movements, and any evidence of seizure-like activity. Sensory testing is often challenging and primarily consists of assessing the patient's response to noxious stimulation. Coordination can be estimated by watching the patient reach for objects if unable to follow more complex commands. Gait should only be assessed if safe to do so.

Serum testing should include a complete metabolic panel, CBC, thyroid studies, and ammonia. These studies may point toward underlying electrolyte disturbances, infection, dehydration, uremic or hepatic encephalopathy, hypoxia, or hypercarbia. Urinalysis, urine culture and urine toxicology should also be obtained. Chest x-ray can uncover a lung infection. A head CT should be considered as several vascular disorders could cause confusion, including ischemic stroke, subdural hemorrhage, subarachnoid hemorrhage, and intracerebral hemorrhage. Even in a patient without a neurological history, a head CT or brain MRI may be warranted if there is no obvious abnormality on initial testing or if the examination uncovers a focal finding. If the mental status continues to fluctuate, an EEG may be needed to rule out nonconvulsive status epilepticus. It is also reasonable to empirically treat for Wernicke's encephalopathy with thiamine 500 mg IV every 8 hours for 3 days, followed by 100 mg/d orally.

In this patient, his lab testing showed a leukocytosis, which was ultimately explained by his steroid use rather than infection. On head CT, the edema around his GBM was mildly improved, as expected with the steroid use. Given his recent seizure, an EEG was obtained, which did not show any further seizures. He was ultimately diagnosed with delirium.

Delirium is an acute change in mental status, characterized by fluctuations in attention and cognition. Delirium is common in the hospital and can affect 10% of general medical admissions and 80% of intensive care unit admissions. While delirium may indicate an underlying life-threatening illness, delirium itself is a serious condition that is associated with several poor clinical outcomes. Even when correcting for illness severity, delirious patients are more likely to stay in the hospital longer, be discharged to nursing homes, and have a higher rate of mortality: two-fold higher than adults who do not develop delirium. The development of delirium is also an independent risk factor for the development of new functional and cognitive decline.

While delirious patients can become agitated (hyperactive delirium), they may also become more lethargic or withdrawn (hypoactive delirium) or show a combination of features (mixed); hypoactive delirium is more likely to be missed.

While antipsychotics, such as Seroquel, were once routinely given to delirious patients, this is no longer recommended unless the patient is a danger to self or others. Rather, the underlying cause of delirium should first be identified. While there are nonmodifiable risk factors for delirium, such as advanced age and cognitive impairment, many other risk factors can be corrected. For instance, hearing or vision impairment can be improved with pocket amplifiers and ensuring glasses are always accessible. If possible, having a family member or a friend at the bedside can help with reorientation and engagement. Immobilization can be corrected by using a safety attendant rather than physical restraints, and tethers, such as urinary catheters—which also carry an infection risk—should be discontinued as soon as possible. Reviewing medications and discontinuing the unnecessary ones can ameliorate polypharmacy. Underlying infection and metabolic derangements should be identified and treated. Adequate sleep is very important but often difficult to achieve in the hospital. Normalization of sleep-wake cycle can make a difference for both prevention and treatment of delirium, and so it is worth reducing the frequency of vital sign checks (if safe to do so), providing ear plugs and an eye mask, and using melatonin (3–10 mg) at night, ensuring pain and nausea are controlled, as well as getting adequate light exposure and avoiding napping during the day (Box 8.1).

BOX 8.1 **Approach to hospital-acquired delirium**

Step 1: Assess airway, breathing, circulation, vital signs, blood glucose. Consider naloxone.

Step 2: Review medications and infection risk factors. Identify signs of infection on exam, perform attention tasks, and look for any focal finding on the neurologic exam.

Obtain BMP, Ca/Mg/Phos, CBC, LFTs, ammonia, VBG, blood cultures, UA, Utox, CXR, EKG.

Step 3: If no obvious cause identified, consider head imaging, EEG, lumbar puncture.

Step 4: If no obvious cause identified, consider thyroid function tests, morning cortisol, vitamin B12, ESR, ANA.

Further Reading

Brown EG, Douglas VC. Moving beyond metabolic encephalopathy: an update on delirium prevention, workup, and management. *Semin Neurol.* 2015;35(6):646–655.

Ely EW, Shintani A, Truman B, et al. Delirium as a predictor of mortality in mechanically ventilated patients in the intensive care unit. *JAMA.* 2004;291(14):1753–1762.

Inouye SK, van Dyck CH, Alessi CA, Balkin S, Siegal AP, Horwitz RI. Clarifying confusion: the confusion assessment method. A new method for detection of delirium. *Ann Intern Med.* 1990;113(12):941–948.

9 Coma with Fever

A 32-year-old man is brought to the hospital when he becomes confused and agitated following a recent camping trip. His temperature is 102°F, blood pressure 104/60 mm Hg, and pulse rate 102. Breathing is regular at a rate of 14. His neck is stiff in flexion/extension but not in rotation. Cardiac auscultation reveals only a soft midsystolic murmur. There is no rash. He is agitated but gradually becomes less responsive. Pupils are 4 mm and react to light equally. Corneal reflexes are intact. Oculocephalic reflex is present. His extremities move sluggishly in response to painful stimulation with some suggestion of decreased power in his right leg. Electrocardiogram is normal. Chest x-ray has not been done yet. Blood count reveals WBC 14,000, RBC 39,000, and electrolytes are normal. Lactate is 4.8. He has been given glucose and naloxone with no response. You are consulted to come and do a lumbar puncture (LP) as the ED staff has tried and failed.

What do you do now?

This seriously ill—perhaps even fatally ill—patient requires quick diagnostic and treatment decision-making. The questions you began considering even on the way to the ED were whether further delay in obtaining CSF is allowable and whether a dangerous mass lesion might be hiding intracranially. The two are connected because puncturing the dura in a patient with increased intracranial pressure, particularly if asymmetrical, as in the case of a temporal mass lesion, could lead to transtentorial herniation, clinical worsening, and even death. So, a head CT is warranted immediately if an LP is needed (which is certainly the case here; see Box 9.1). But there has already been delay and waiting for the CT will add further delay. So, the first step is to lessen the danger here: starting broad-coverage antimicrobial therapy immediately, in addition to steroids, in order to at least begin treating what might be a life-threatening meningitis or encephalitis. Once this is started, proceeding to head CT in a brisk fashion, followed by LP, will be possible. There are several blood tests to keep in mind, including obtaining a CBC, lactate, HIV, and blood cultures. Blood cultures can aid in the diagnosis in a majority of cases and should be obtained before antibiotics are started.

Interestingly, what we were taught in medical school about the nature of meningismus is correct: stiffness in flexion-extension is indicative of meningeal irritation; stiffness in rotation is not. Therefore, this patient clearly has meningismus. Meningitis can be caused by a number of organisms in this age group, and, surprisingly, the relative probability of various organisms has changed somewhat over the past few years, probably as a result of the *H. influenza* and *S. pneumoniae* vaccines. For example, gram-negative

---

BOX 9.1 **When to obtain a head CT before LP**

Age >60 years
History of central nervous system disease
Immunocompromised
New-onset seizure within the past week
Altered mental status or coma
Optic disc edema
Focal neurologic deficit

bacteria and *Staphylococcus* have overtaken *Streptococcus* in some areas as the most common cause.

Despite advances in antibiotic choices and early diagnosis, approximately 10–20% of adults with meningitis will die from it and another similar fraction will have significant morbidity from it. Initial choices in antibiotic therapy should consist of ceftriaxone (2 g IV every 12 hours), vancomycin (1 g IV every eight hours if <65 kg or 1.5 g IV every eight hours if >65 kg), and acyclovir 10 mg/kg every eight hours with the possible addition of ampicillin 2 g IV every four hours if *Listeria monocytogenes* is suspected (e.g., in older or immune-compromised patients). There is growing resistance to even these antibiotics, however, which unfortunately makes culture results even more important. Nosocomial causes of meningitis, as well as suspected meningitis after penetrating head injury, lead to different etiological considerations, which is not an issue with this case.

The addition of corticosteroids before or with initial antibiotics in the management of strongly suspected bacterial meningitis is generally done at a high dose as soon as possible, despite some conflicting evidence of efficacy. A common approach is to use dexamethasone 0.15 mg/kg every six hours IV for 4 days.

The suppressed mental status in this patient is concerning, and so a head CT should be expedited. If possible, CT with contrast can be helpful as it increases the sensitivity for identifying meningeal and intraparenchymal involvement. Cerebral edema may occur in bacterial meningitis, which may cause elevated intracranial pressure and/or hydrocephalus. Certain bacteria, especially *S. pneumoniae*, can lead to vascular complications such as arterial and venous thrombi. For this reason, it is important to also obtain CT angiography and CT venography of the brain when getting the screening head CT.

Measuring an opening pressure with the LP can be helpful if this is abnormally elevated. Legs should be straightened prior to measuring the pressure as bent legs can falsely elevate it.

There should be a Gram stain and culture performed on the CSF. In the presenting case, if this patient does have bacterial meningitis, there may be a problem in identifying the causative organism in culture since antibiotics were begun before CSF obtained. This is another reason why drawing blood cultures before starting antibiotics is so important. Fortunately, for most bacterial causes of meningitis, cultures will be positive even after antibiotics are started. This is less true for *Neisseria*, but for all bacterial causes, Gram stain data will be abnormal for many hours, and neutrophil-prominent pleocytosis will persist as well. Low glucose and high protein will likewise be present for some time after treatment is begun (Table 9.1). If lab evaluation is equivocal, polymerase chain reaction (PCR) testing for common causal organisms may be obtained. Herpes simplex virus 1 and 2 PCR should always be done if there is any chance of viral encephalitis, in addition to varicella zoster virus PCR, IgG, and IgM. It is also reasonable to test for fungi, such as *Cryptococcus*, in the CSF and serum. This patient should also be investigated for other infectious diseases, depending on what is endemic to the area or recent travel history, and head MRI, MR angiography (to assess for possible vasculopathy), and MR venography (to exclude cerebral venous thrombosis) should be considered.

TABLE 9.1 **CSF patterns in meningitis of various etiologies**

Pathogen	CSF differential	CSF glucose	CSF protein
Bacterial	PMNs (may be lymphocytic if partially treated)	Low	High
Viral	Lymphocytic (PMNs may present acutely)	Normal	Normal/High
Mycobacterial	Lymphocytic	Low	High
Fungal	Lymphocytic (some may be more monocytic)	Low	Normal/High
CNS lymphoma, carcinomatous	Abnormal cells, mononuclear	Normal/Low	High
T. solium, C. immitis, Angiostrongyluscantonensis, Gnathostoma, hardware	Eosinophils		
CMV, EBV, enterovirus, VZV, WNV	Atypical lymphocytes		

Patients with suspected bacterial meningitis should be placed in respiratory isolation for the first day of treatment if possible until the organism is identified. Patients with meningococcal meningitis should remain on droplet precautions for at least 24 hours after antibiotics are begun, although specific guidelines vary by hospital. Pneumococcal and viral causes do not require isolation. Meningococcal meningitis contacts should be treated prophylactically once the organism is identified depending on local policy.

There are several complications to remain vigilant for if your patient is not improving. Meningitis may result in hydrocephalus due to reduced CSF absorption, or cerebral edema, which may require placement of an extraventricular drain or use of hyperosmolar agents like mannitol or hypertonic saline. Lack of source control may cause worsening, and so a search for a parameningeal focus, such as an epidural abscess, may be warranted. These patients are also at increased risk for seizure, including nonconvulsive status epilepticus, so EEG should be considered if mental status remains poor.

KEY POINTS TO REMEMBER

- Bacterial meningitis must be treated with a broad-coverage antibiotic regimen as soon as possible to prevent morbidity and mortality, even if this means treating prior to obtaining CSF.
- Bacterial blood cultures should be obtained before giving antibiotics.
- CSF Gram stain and white blood cell results remain abnormal for many hours following the initiation of antibiotics.
- Corticosteroids have been shown to be effective in reducing rates of hearing loss and neurological complications in patients with meningitis due to *S. pneumoniae* and should be given in addition to antibiotics.
- Bacterial meningitis may lead to arterial and venous clots, and so vessel imaging should be obtained for any focal neurologic exam finding or suppressed mental status.

Further Reading

Durand ML, Calderwood SB, Weber DJ, Miller SI, Southwick, Caviness VS, Swartz
    MN. Acute bacterial meningitis in adults: a review of 493 episodes. *N Engl J Med.*
    1993;328:21–28.

Hasbun R, Abrahams J, Jekel J, et al. Computed tomography of the head
    before lumbar puncture in adults with suspected meningitis. *N Engl J Med.*
    2001;345(24):1727–1733.

Tunkel AR, Hartman BJ, Kaplan SL, et al. Practice guidelines for the management of
    bacterial meningitis. *Clin Infect Dis.* 2004;39(9):1267–1284.

10 Refractory Vertigo

A 65-year-old woman is seen in the ED for severe dizziness for the past 3 days. She relates brief milder episodes of this in the past. She has vomited, has a mild headache posteriorly, and states she is unable to walk. She endorses a sensation of "things moving" and not knowing "which way is up." She denies vision changes, trouble speaking, sensory changes, and weakness. Her medical history is remarkable for hypertension and pre-diabetes. She had migraine headaches in her 20s. General exam is normal. Neurological exam is remarkable for midposition poorly reactive pupils and horizontal nystagmus, worse on gaze to the left. Her speech is slightly dysarthric. Strength is normal. Reflexes are diffusely diminished. Touch and proprioception are slightly reduced in her feet. Gait is unsteady, but base is not widened. CT scan of the head reveals some cortical atrophy and subtle white matter changes bilaterally.

What do you do now?

Sorting out the patient with "dizziness" can be tricky. The first step in evaluating these patients is to distinguish between the major symptoms which can lead a patient to complain of dizziness: (1) vertigo, (2) lightheadedness and (3) disequilibrium. This can be more difficult than expected since these perceptions do overlap, and particularly if your patient has any degree of mental fogginess or anxiety (not uncommon). And of course, there are a number of patients who use the word "dizzy" to refer to other perceptions like confusion, visual change, clumsiness or even anxiety.

Patients using the words "unbalanced", "wobbly", and "unsteady" are generally describing disequilibrium, which usually implicates cerebellar, cortico-cerebellar connections, or dorsal column sensory dysfunction. CT scan of the head is a good initial step here, to rule out brainstem or cerebellar hemorrhage. An acute brainstem or cerebellar stroke will not be seen, so MRI is necessary to discover this. Generally, cerebrovascular causes of vertigo or imbalance will be accompanied by other signs of ischemia. A common cerebrovascular cause of vertigo is the Wallenberg syndrome, due to lateral medullary ischemia, which can consist of dysphagia, slurred speech, ataxia, ipsilateral facial sensation loss, contralateral body sensation loss, vertigo, nystagmus, Horner's syndrome, and diplopia. In some cases, ataxia and vertigo do predominate. A special case, vertebral dissection, can lead to ischemia of the brainstem with prominent balance issues, along with headache which tends to be posterior in location but may radiate anteriorly as well.

Lightheadedness is usually the term patients choose to describe presyncope, which is generally related to some reduction in cerebral perfusion. This can be due to any number of conditions from dehydration to a serious cardiovascular condition (see Chapter 9 - Syncope). Workup should begin with a thorough cardiovascular exam and an ECG. More lengthy cardiac monitoring, echocardiography, and imaging of the cervical arteries with CT or MRI angiography may be necessary as well. Tilt table testing may be indicated if autonomic instability is suspected.

Patients who describe a sensation of movement are probably feeling vertiginous, which implicates a lesion or lesions in labyrinths, vestibular nerves, or vestibular brainstem centers. Nausea is usually an accompaniment. Vestibular neuronitis or "labyrinthitis", thought to be a self-limited viral or otherwise inflammatory reaction in the labyrinthine system, is a common cause of vertigo at all ages. Bacterial infections of the middle ear can also lead to vertigo along with hearing changes. Benign positional vertigo, thought to be due to otolith formation within the semicircular canals, should not be prolonged as in this patient and positional triggering is usually described by the patient. In all of these cases of so-called "peripheral" vertigo (stemming from labyrinthine or vestibular nerve pathology) imaging will be negative but the Dix-Hallpike maneuver should be positive with induction of severe vertigo (and probably nausea) when the extended head is turned to the side of the dysfunctional inner ear in the supine position. In addition, nystagmus (generally horizontal or diagonal, not vertical) is brought on by this maneuver, but this can vary.

Meniere's disease, thought to result from chronic excess endolymph in inner ear structures, is eventually accompanied by hearing loss and/or tinnitus, but may not yet be present initially. Perilymph fistula also generally involves a hearing loss, and there is almost always a history of a prior incident like weightlifting, barotrauma, scuba diving, or forceful nose-blowing. Meningeal infection or inflammation is usually suggested by meningismus, headache, other cranial neuropathies. Superior semicircular canal dehiscence can cause new and persistent vertigo, with clues to diagnosis including sound induced vertigo, hyperacusis and vertigo.

In migraine-related vertigo—aka vestibular migraine (VM)—there is usually a history of migraine, or at least a strong family history, coupling of symptoms with headache at least some of the time, and response to migraine abortive medications (like triptans). The mechanism of vertigo in migraine may relate to the many interconnections between vestibular and head pain networks or perhaps to the overall sensory "disintegration" postulated in migraine. There is some belief in a form of VM that generally is independent of head pain and can occur episodically on its own. A relatively new entity—*persistent postural perceptual vertigo* PPPV—is currently not well understood but is diagnosed when the following triad is present: persistent subjective non-rotational vertigo or dizziness, hypersensitivity to motion stimuli (self or surroundings), and difficulties with visual tasks. Typically, these patients have normal clinical balance tests, and there are no vestibular tests which diagnose them with accuracy. The mechanism of PPPV is unclear but seems to be based on multisensory dysfunction in integrating vestibular, visual and motion stimuli in the CNS.

Psychogenic vertigo does occur, but one might expect an absence of nystagmus and other neurological signs and a history of phobias or panic attacks. A number of medications can produce vertigo including antiarrhythmics, antihypertensives, antihistamines, amphetamines, antimicrobials, digoxin, muscle relaxants, bladder control anticholinergics, lithium, and antiparkinson medications.

Vestibular nerve involvement may be due to a mass in the cerebellopontine angle or an infectious/inflammatory process in the subarachnoid space affecting the acoustic nerve. Hence MRI and lumbar puncture are indicated if suspicion is high, particularly if other focal findings are seen on exam such as cranial neuropathies. Lyme titer, angiotensin converting enzyme level, and VDRL are all worth considering in these cases. Electronystagmography may eventually confirm a labyrinthine cause of vertigo, but even then, cerebrovascular etiology is not entirely ruled out since small vessel embolization (to the internal auditory artery, or vestibular artery) or other occlusive pathophysiology can lead to similar results with essentially isolated vertigo.

A helpful diagnostic exercise can be to try to determine whether vertigo is "peripheral" (due to labyrinthine or vestibular nerve dysfunction) or "central" (brainstem or cerebral causes). Much study has been devoted to making this determination, but it remains challenging. Kattah et al. in 2009 found that a battery of three bedside tests had good accuracy in differentiating posterior circulation stroke from peripheral vestibulopathy, details of which are outlined in their article in the suggested reading list at the end of this chapter. (Box 10.1 provides a full list of the causes of isolated vertigo.)

This patient seems to have isolated new onset vertigo, with similar episodes in the past. Her accompanying symptoms and signs of nausea and walking difficulty seem attributable to the vertigo itself. The pupillary unreactivity is probably related to cataract surgery, and the distal sensation loss may very well be due to diabetic peripheral neuropathy. So, a labyrinthine cause of vertigo, such as vestibular neuronitis or a central cause, particularly vestibular migraine, are both high on the list. But she has risk factors for stroke and is in an age group where this is more probable—so she should probably be admitted at least for observation while workup is pending. One should be prepared for

BOX 10.1 **Causes of isolated vertigo**

Labyrinthine or vestibular nerve dysfunction:

Benign Positional Vertigo

Medication effect – aspirin, nonsteroidal anti-inflammatory drugs, phenytoin, aminoglycosides

Vestibular neuronitis/Labyrinthitis

Meniere's disease

Post-traumatic vertigo

Cogan's syndrome – Autoimmune disease of inner ear

Arnold Chiari syndrome

Neurosyphilis – labyrinth infection, meningitis, arteritis

Intralabyrinthine hemorrhage (leukemia, trauma)

Sarcoidosis

Perilymph fistula

Meningitis – Carcinomatous, TB, fungal, bacterial

Ramsay Hunt syndrome (Zoster infection of Geniculate ganglion)

Labyrinthine ischemia

CNS causes

Brainstem or cerebellopontine region tumor

Brainstem or cerebellar ischemia

Brainstem AVM

Complex partial seizures

Migraine

MS – brainstem plaque

Brainstem neoplasm

Hyperventilation

Hypothyroidism

Hypoglycemia

Carcinoid syndrome

Cardiac arrhythmia

Pheochromocytoma

Phobic vertigo

a negative workup however, since cerebrovascular causes of isolated vertigo are actually infrequent.

Despite the cause, vertigo can be treated with anticholinergics or antihistamines reasonably well. Many patients find oral or parenteral hydroxyzine 25–50 mg to be helpful, and for severe vertigo, transdermal scopolamine is often very effective. Vertigo and associated nausea or vomiting can be treated with a neuroleptic class antiemetic such as promethazine 25 mg IV. Benzodiazepine medication such as lorazepam 1–2 mg IV is quite helpful acutely. Although systemic corticosteroids have been recommended as a treatment for vestibular neuritis, there is insufficient evidence. If migrainous vertigo is suspected, a trial of a triptan (if cerebro- and cardiovascular disease has been ruled out) may be very useful. And perhaps preventive meds such as a beta blocker, tricyclic antidepressant, or topiramate might be of use.

KEY POINTS TO REMEMBER

- "Dizziness" can indicate any of several different states including vertigo, imbalance, and lightheadedness, with significant perceptual overlap.
- In patients who have risk factors for cardiovascular and cerebrovascular disease, an initial CT scan, and later MRI, cerebral vascular imaging, and echocardiography are probably indicated.
- Vertigo when accompanied by cranial neuropathies should prompt LP, after head imaging, if there are no contraindications.
- Significant lightheadedness with or without syncope should lead to cardiac evaluation.

Further Reading

Grad A, Baloh RW. Vertigo of vascular origin: clinical and electronystagmographic features in 84 cases. *Arch Neurol.* 1989;46:281–284.

Huang TC, Wang SJ, Kheradman A. Vestibular migraine: an update on current understanding and future directions. *Cephalalgia.* 2020;40:107–121.

Kattah JC, Talkad AV, Wang DZ, et al. HINTS to diagnose stroke in the acute vestibular syndrome. *Stroke.* 2009;40:3504–3510.

Kerber KA, Brown DL, Lisabeth LD, et al. Stroke among patients with dizziness, vertigo, and imbalance in the emergency department: a population-based study. *Stroke.* 2006;37:2484–2487.

11   Febrile Dystonia

A 35-year-old man was brought to the ED
from a drug and alcohol rehabilitation facility
because of abnormal movements and a change
in behavior. He carries the diagnoses of bipolar
affective disorder and alcohol/sedative use
disorder. His current medication list includes
fluoxetine, olanzapine, and nortriptyline. His
temperature is 40°C and his blood pressure is
160/100. He is tachycardic at 120. Mental status is
initially remarkable for some mild agitation, but,
over time, he becomes somnolent. Neurological
exam reveals a mild action tremor, occasional
myoclonic jerks in his lower extremities,
hyperactive muscle stretch reflexes, ankle
clonus, and diffusely increased muscle tone.
White blood cell count is normal at 10,000.
Creatine kinase (CK) is mildly elevated at 550 U/
L. Chemistry panel is otherwise normal. Urine
toxicology is pending.

What do you do now?

The initial step in patients with fever and altered mental status is to rule out life-threatening CNS infection. After plain CT is negative for a mass lesion or hemorrhage, lumbar puncture (LP) will help to rule out meningitis and encephalitis. There are occasional cases of viral encephalitis with benign CSF, and if suspicion is high, initiating antiviral therapy while awaiting polymerase chain reaction (PCR) testing results for herpes simplex virus (HSV) and varicella zoster virus (VZV) might be reasonable. Status epilepticus is another possibility here but is unlikely with his relatively preserved mental status exam (EEG may be necessary when there is a question). Once workup has ruled these out, a number of possibilities present themselves here, each requiring a different management approach.

His medication regimen suggests the possibility of a drug-induced syndrome such as neuroleptic malignant syndrome (NMS), serotonin syndrome (SS), or anticholinergic toxicity. And just because he is in a rehab center, it should not be assumed that he is not intoxicated or withdrawing from a substance. Alcohol withdrawal in particular can mimic many medication-induced symptoms. Urine toxicology will exclude substance intoxication but not a withdrawal syndrome. A vague history concerning medications and doses adds to the challenge, of course, and one must always consider that patients have used higher doses than prescribed and the possibility of other drug use. Drugs like cocaine and amphetamines (including methylenedioxymethamphetamine [MDMA]) can produce an encephalopathy, though fever and myoclonus is not typical.

Neuroleptic medications can induce several neurological syndromes: (1) acute dystonia, (2) akathisia, (3) oculogyric crisis, (4) parkinsonism, (5) tardive dyskinesia, and (6) NMS. This patient's presentation is in some ways typical for NMS—encephalopathy, hyperthermia, muscle rigidity, tachycardia—but the CK level is not as high as is typical in NMS. This patient could be early in the development of the NMS syndrome, so CK should be rechecked. It is not unreasonable to begin treatment presumptively in suspicious cases. Treatment consists of cooling, dantrolene sodium (a direct acting muscle relaxant) 1–2 mg/kg IV, repeated every few hours, and bromocriptine 2.5–10 mg three times a day. Volume depletion must be corrected with IV fluids. Hypotension may also respond to fluid boluses. Cooling methods include cooling blankets, ice packs, cold IV fluids, and antipyretics. When rhabdomyolysis occurs, hydration and alkalinization of the urine with sodium bicarbonate is essential in hopes of preventing renal failure. Benzodiazepines can also help reduce muscle rigidity. Prognosis in NMS was said to be poor in the past, but, more recently, with proper care, at least 90% of patients will survive.

The viral encephalitis of rabies resembles NMS a bit more than does HSV or the other viral encephalitides. Patients can present with the "furious" form with fever, agitation, motor hyperactivity, hallucinosis, confusion, and, ultimately, seizures and coma. There can be calm (lucid) periods. Rigidity is unlikely, although sometimes there can be motor weakness. While it is uncommon to contract rabies from an infected human, precautions must be observed if it is suspected.

Anti-NMDA receptor encephalitis can present with abnormal movements (generally seizures at some point) and fever, and it is diagnosed with autoantibody testing from blood and CSF samples.

Malignant hyperthermia is a genetic disorder resulting from ryanodine receptor mutations, which presents with fever, rigidity, tremors, agitated delirium, and hallucinosis, and progresses to stupor and coma. It is generally provoked by inhalational anesthetics and/or depolarizing muscle relaxants. Treatment consists of cooling, dantrolene sodium 1–2 mg/kg IV, in repeated doses, and bicarbonate to normalize metabolic acidosis. Arrhythmias must be treated and electrolyte imbalances corrected. It can be difficult to differentiate from NMS, so history is crucial.

Overdose with anticholinergic medication including cyclic antidepressants and antihistamines can present with febrile encephalopathy. The presentation can include fever, tachycardia, hypotension, encephalopathy, and muscle rigidity. Skin is usually dry, and the patient has mydriasis.

Serotonin syndrome (SS), due usually to additive effects of multiple serotonergic medications, seems the most likely diagnosis here. SS is usually accompanied by hyperreflexia, as opposed to the hyporeflexia seen with NMS. Also, patients with SS typically have a normal WBC count. Medications that may contribute to excessive serotonin effect via various mechanisms include tricyclic antidepressants, selective serotonin reuptake inhibitors (SSRIs), serotonin-norepinephrine reuptake inhibitors (SNRIs), buspirone, the serotonin-3 receptor antagonists (e.g., ondansetron), dextromethorphan, carbamazepine, valproate, cyclobenzaprine, metoclopramide, tramadol, monoamine oxidase inhibitors (MAOIs), ergot derivatives (including LSD), and lithium.

Treatment of SS should, of course, include discontinuation of all serotonergic agents. In mild cases, symptoms resolve within a day or two at most. Cooling agents, antihypertensives, nasal oxygen, and benzodiazepines can all be helpful. Those with severe symptoms, including autonomic instability not responsive to initial therapies, may warrant treatment with the serotonin blocker cyproheptadine. Patients who are severely hyperthermic or agitated might need endotracheal intubation to support respiration and to protect their airway as the serotonin effect wanes.

The diagnosis in cases of delirium with hyperthermia, like the one presenting here, can be challenging, with overlapping symptoms and signs seen in several conditions (Box 11.1 and Table 11.1). A menu of testing includes CT of the head, LP with CSF analysis including viral PCR testing, EEG, CBC, full chemistry panel, toxicology screen, urine myoglobin, lactate and CK levels, arterial blood gases, and blood cultures.

TABLE 11.1 **Comparison of presentation in serotonin syndrome (SS), neuroleptic malignant syndrome (NMS), malignant hyperthermia, and anticholinergic overdose**

Symptom/ sign	Serotonin syndrome	NMS	Malignant hyperthermia	Anticholinergic toxicity
Delirium	+	+	+	+
Fever	+	+	+	+
Autonomic dysfunction	+	+	+	+
Pupils	Dilated			Dilated
Nausea/ Vomiting	+			
Rigidity	+	++	+	+
Reflexes	Increased	Decreased	Decreased	
Myoclonus	+			
Tremor	+			
CK	Increased	High	High	
Treatment	Benzodiazepine, cyproheptadine, antihistamine	Bromocriptine, dantrolene, benzodiazepine	Dantrolene	

KEY POINTS TO REMEMBER

- Febrile encephalopathy is a dire emergency that requires a speedy workup and possibly empiric antibiotic treatment while diagnostic tests are pending.
- Muscle rigidity, sympathetic lability, high CK and febrile encephalopathy, in the context of dopamine antagonist use or dopamine agonist withdrawal, are suggestive of NMS.
- Myoclonic jerks and hyperreflexia are more typical of SS.

Further Reading

Ables AZ, Nagubilli R. Prevention, recognition, and management of serotonin syndrome. *Am Fam Physician*. 2010;1;81:1139–1142.

Broderick ED, Crosby B. Anticholinergic toxicity. 2018;StatPearls [Internet].

Gillman KP. Triptans, serotonin agonists, and serotonin syndrome (serotonin toxicity): a review. *Headache: The Journal of Head and Face Pain*, 2010;50:264–272.

Turner AH, Kim JJ, McCarron RM, Nguyen CT. Differentiating serotonin syndrome and neuroleptic malignant syndrome. *Current Psychiatry*. 2016;18:30–36.

Werneke U, Jamshidi F, Taylor D, et al. Conundrums in neurology: diagnosing serotonin syndrome: a metaanalysis of cases. *BMC Neurol*. 2016;16:97.

12 Myelopathy

A 70-year-old painter with history of metastatic colon cancer presents with progressive weakness and numbness in his hands over the course of a week. He reports difficulty with holding paint brushes and yesterday recognized a new imbalance and weakness in his legs. He denies incontinence or constipation. His vital signs are unremarkable with a blood pressure of 130/70 and heart rate of 70; he is afebrile. He appears well on his general physical exam. His mental status is intact, and he has no cranial nerve deficits. His finger taps are slowed bilaterally; his foot taps are also mildly slowed. He has reduced vibration in the feet but no clear sensory level to pinprick. He is hyperreflexic in the legs. He underwent an MRI of the cervical spine showing a long segment of abnormal signal in the cervical cord as well as an area with contrast enhancement.

What do you do now?

A detailed history is helpful here as we think about localization and cause. First, clarify the onset of symptoms. Weakness that occurs acutely may be due to structural diseases of the spinal cord or vascular causes (e.g., ischemic stroke, hemorrhage). Subacute myelopathy is more likely to be due to infection or autoimmune/inflammatory diseases or tumors. Subacute to chronic myelopathies may be due to neurodegenerative diseases, infections such as HIV or human T-lymphotropic virus (HTLV), metabolic derangements, or insidious compression from a structural cause. Is the weakness static, relapsing, or progressive? Are there any predisposing factors, such as trauma, recent illness, or toxic exposures? Determining if there is additional involvement of the face, arms, bowel/bladder function, or asymmetrical weakness can aid with localization. In addition to weakness, is there pain or numbness, and if so, where?

The localization of bilateral leg weakness is broad. Before focusing on the spinal cord, it is a helpful exercise to think of all the other possibilities. Another CNS cause is from a rare variant of the anterior cerebral artery (ACA), called the *azygos ACA*. Diseases affecting multiple nerve roots (polyradiculopathy), including at the level of the cauda equina (cauda equina syndrome), may result in bilateral leg weakness. Bilateral lumbosacral plexopathy, such as from diabetic amyotrophy, may have pain, muscle atrophy, and weakness. Diseases that affect multiple peripheral nerves, such as Guillain-Barré syndrome, can cause bilateral leg weakness that is often asymmetrical. A variety of diseases (e.g., myasthenia gravis, botulism) can affect the neuromuscular junction, which can cause bilateral leg weakness but may also affect bulbar musculature, too. Last, diseases that affect the muscle, such as inclusion body myositis, are more likely to affect the proximal musculature of the leg.

The first goal for any suspected myelopathy is to rule out a compressive cause, which may require urgent surgical treatment (Box 12.1). Compression can be due to trauma, degenerative spine disease, infection (e.g., epidural abscess, tuberculosis infection of the vertebral bodies), neoplasm (e.g., meningioma, metastasis), or other abnormalities within the epidural space, such as lipomatosis or hemorrhage. Identifying the presence of a compression often requires imaging, preferably MRI. Flexion-extension x-rays also allow for detection of dynamic instability of the vertebral bodies.

Compressive myelopathy causes

- Trauma
- Degenerative spine disease
- Infection
  • Epidural abscess, TB of the vertebral bodies
- Neoplastic
  • Meningioma, metastasis
- Other
  • Fatty infiltration of the epidural space (lipomatosis), hemorrhage

Noncompressive myelopathy causes

- Noninflammatory
  • Neoplastic
  • Lymphoma, glioma
  • Toxic/Metabolic
  • Intrathecal chemotherapy, post-radiation
  • Vitamin/mineral deficiency: vitamin B12, vitamin E, copper
  • Vascular
  • Ischemic stroke, AVM, dAVF
  • Genetic
  • Friedreich ataxia, hereditary spastic paraplegia, adrenoleukodystrophy spinocerebellar ataxia, amyotrophic lateral sclerosis
- Inflammatory
  • Autoimmune/demyelinating
  • CNS: MS, NMO, MOG
  • Systemic: SLE, Sjögren's, sarcoidosis, vasculitis
  • Infectious
  • Bacterial: TB, Syphilis
  • Viral: Herpes viruses (HSV, VZV, EBV, CMV), HIV, HTLV; Enterovirus, WNV
  • Parasitic: Schistosoma
  • Paraneoplastic
  • Anti-Hu, anti-CRMP5, anti-amphiphysin

Noncompressive myelopathy can be neoplastic, vascular, toxic/metabolic, genetic, or inflammatory. Neoplastic causes include lymphoma as well as primary spinal cord tumors such as a glioma. Vascular causes include ischemic infarcts, such as to the anterior spinal artery, leading to an anterior cord syndrome (deficits in motor and spinothalamic tract but preservation of dorsal column function) or the presence of a vascular malformation, such as arteriovenous malformation (AVM) or dural arteriovenous fistula (dAVF). Spinal dAVF are especially important to have on the differential for an older man with a slowly progressive myelopathy—carefully look at the MRI for the presence of flow voids.

The identification of a toxic/metabolic etiology can be aided by a thorough history, including medications, prior surgeries (e.g., gastric bypass), and health-related behaviors, such as the use of nitrous oxide canister "whippits". Intrathecal chemotherapy may be a toxic source of myelopathy. Exposure of the spinal cord to radiation may produce early delayed (within 6 months) or delayed (years later) radiation myelopathy. Metabolic causes include vitamin B12 deficiency, functional vitamin B12 deficiency due to nitrous oxide exposure, vitamin E deficiency, or copper deficiency (which can be from zinc excess: watch out for denture cream!). Decompression sickness, a complication of scuba diving, can result immediately or within days of ascent, often affecting the thoracic cord.

There are several genetic disorders associated with myelopathy, including Friedreich ataxia, hereditary spastic paraplegia, and adrenoleukodystrophy. Spinocerebellar ataxia is an autosomal dominant disease that may feature myelopathy in addition to ataxia. Amyotrophic lateral sclerosis usually has mixed upper and lower motor neuron signs but can present with myelopathy.

The main categories of inflammatory myelopathy (myelitis) are autoimmune/demyelinating, infectious, and paraneoplastic. There are several autoimmune diseases that affect the CNS. These include multiple sclerosis, neuromyelitis optica spectrum disorder (NMOSD), and myelin oligodendrocyte glycoprotein antibody (anti-MOG). Clues for NMOSD include the presence of a longitudinally extensive spinal cord lesion that extends for at least three vertebral segments. The presence of NMO-IgG in serum is supportive of this diagnosis. CSF may feature a neutrophilic pleocytosis, and oligoclonal bands are often absent. Anti-MOG can be distinguished from NMOSD as these cases are more likely to present with simultaneous bilateral optic neuritis and have fewer relapses, and the spinal cord lesions may be more likely to occur in the lower regions of the spinal cord. The presence of MOG-IgG is supportive.

Systemic autoimmune diseases that can result in myelopathy include systemic lupus erythematous, sarcoidosis, Sjögren's syndrome, and vasculitis.

There are several infectious causes of noncompressive myelitis. Viruses are the most common pathogen and include the herpes viruses (herpes simplex virus, varicella zoster virus, Epstein Barr virus, and human cytomegalovirus), hepatitis C virus, HIV-associated vacuolar myelopathy, and HTLV-I. Certain viruses can also affect the anterior horn cells resulting in flaccid weakness and absent reflexes. These viruses include enteroviruses (e.g., poliovirus, coxsackie virus) and the flaviviruses (e.g., West Nile virus and Japanese encephalitis virus). In addition to causing a compressive myelopathy (Pott's disease), tuberculosis can cause tuberculomas that also cause myelopathy. Syphilis primarily affects the dorsal columns. The parasite *Schistosoma* more often affects the thoracic spinal cord and can result in symptoms of transverse myelitis; here, CSF may show a pleocytosis with eosinophilia.

While rarer, there are paraneoplastic causes for myelopathy. These are thought to be due to an autoimmune reaction to an antigen shared by a tumor. The most common example is anti-Hu, which is associated with breast and lung cancers. Antibodies to amphiphysin, collapsin response-mediator protein-5 (CRMP5), and glutamic acid decarboxylase (GAD) may also present with myelopathy.

So many things can result in myelopathy! How to narrow the differential? After obtaining a detailed history and physical exam, spinal cord imaging is the next step, such as an MRI with and without contrast (see Figures 12.1 and 12.2). Presence of a sensory level can help guide which spinal cord segment should be imaged first. It is also reasonable to obtain an MRI of the brain if there is any possibility that the localization is not specific to the spinal cord. If there is concern for a vascular malformation, then a conventional angiogram will be needed for diagnosis and treatment. Otherwise, if trying to determine if the myelopathy is inflammatory or noninflammatory, serum studies assessing for the causes outlined earlier, as well as CSF sampling, is necessary.

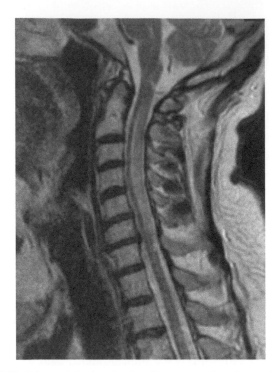

FIGURE 12.1   MRI of the cervical spine showing a long segment hyperintense intramedullary central cervical cord lesion.

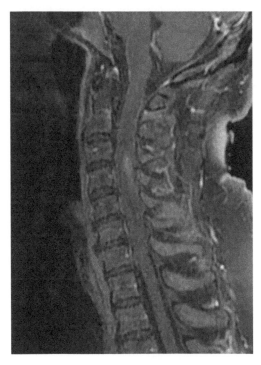

FIGURE 12.2   MRI of the same cervical spine lesion as in Figure 12.1, but with enhancement.

While carrying out the diagnostic work-up, it is important to remember management of complications that can arise from myelopathy, such as checking a post-void residual to assess for urinary retention, and DVT prophylaxis if mobility is limited.

KEY POINTS TO REMEMBER

- If someone presents with a myelopathy, the first goal is to determine if it is from a compression to the spinal cord.
- Flexion-extension x-rays can help identify dynamic instability that may result in intermittent cord compression.
- Once compression is ruled out, consider differentiating inflammatory from noninflammatory causes of myelopathy, which often requires CSF analysis.
- Remain vigilant for vascular causes of myelopathy, including the presence of a spinal dural arteriovenous fistula.

Further Reading

Barreras P, Fitzgerald KC, Mealy MA, et al. Clinical biomarkers differentiate myelitis from vascular and other causes of myelopathy. *Neurology.* 2018;90(1):e12–e21.

Cho TA, Bhattacharyya S. Approach to myelopathy. *Continuum (Minneap Minn).* 2018;24(2, Spinal Cord Disorders):386–406.

Graber JJ, Nolan CP. Myelopathics in patients with cancer. *Arch Neurol.* 2010;67(3):298–304.

13 Neurologic Complications of Immune Checkpoint Inhibitors

A 43-year-old man is admitted for aspiration pneumonia. He has a history of nasopharyngeal carcinoma treated with radiation, chemotherapy, and resection. He started pembrolizumab several months ago without progression of his cancer. On admission, he required 3 L oxygen via nasal cannula but had otherwise normal vital signs. He now complains of difficulty keeping his head up. His voice has become quieter, and he has difficulty swallowing. He denies diplopia but endorses generalized weakness. When you examine him in the afternoon, his mental status is normal. His speech is hypophonic and dysarthric. Pupils are symmetric and reactive. There is bilateral ptosis that worsens with sustained upgaze. Extraocular movements are full. There is weakness of neck flexion and deltoids; the remainder of the muscle groups are full strength. Sensation and reflexes are intact throughout. When you examine him the next morning, his ptosis is improved, and his voice is clearer.

What do you do now?

The neurologic exam of this patient features several findings that are suspicious for a process beyond local involvement of the cancer. The combination of ocular, bulbar, neck, and proximal limb weakness may localize to the subarachnoid space affecting multiple roots, the neuromuscular junction, or muscles. The fluctuation of the weakness and absence of sensory deficits is most concerning for a neuromuscular junction disorder, such as myasthenia gravis. This patient's chest pain and dyspnea may be from a concomitant myocarditis or myositis affecting the muscles of respiration.

One key piece of history is the use of pembrolizumab, an immune checkpoint inhibitor (ICPi). Initially approved for metastatic melanoma, ICPis are increasingly used for the treatment of many types of cancers. ICPis are monoclonal antibodies that block the checkpoint pathways that normally dampen the immune system, enabling T-cells to attack cancer cells. The current FDA-approved ICPis fall into three classes: anti-CTLA-4 (ipilimumab), anti-PD-1 (nivolumab, pembrolizumab), and anti-PDL-1 (atezolizumab, avelumab, durvalumab).

While a groundbreaking cancer treatment, inhibition of immune checkpoints can lead to *immune-related adverse events* (irAEs) that can affect any organ system and are more common when ICPis from different classes are used in combination. While irAEs are more likely to develop 8–12 weeks from treatment start, they can be idiosyncratic to the start of the drug. Neurologic irAEs occur in approximately 1–4% of patients treated with ICPis and affect the peripheral nervous system twice as often as the central nervous system. Examples of irAEs include encephalitis; aseptic meningitis; transverse myelitis; axonal or demyelinating neuropathy affecting motor, sensory, or autonomic nerves; disorders of the neuromuscular junction, such as myasthenia gravis or Lambert-Eaton myasthenic syndrome (LEMS); and myositis.

The severity of irAEs, distinguished by toxicity "grades," is variable. While rare, neurologic irAEs have a higher risk of fatality than other irAEs. For this reason, it is important to be vigilant for such complications when caring for a patient exposed to one of these medications. While the reason for these complications is not fully understood, possibilities include increased T-cell activity against both cancerous and host tissue, increased levels of preexisting autoantibodies, and heightened inflammation. The most comprehensive guidelines on the management of irAEs were published by the American Society of Clinical Oncology.

Symptoms of myasthenia gravis in the setting of ICPi use may overlap with myositis, myocarditis, or thyroiditis. The workup includes pulmonary function testing, especially forced vital capacity (FVC) and mean inspiratory force (MIF), and several blood tests, including creatinine kinase, thyroid-stimulating hormone (TSH), and free T4, as well as acetylcholine receptor (AChR) and antistriated muscle antibodies. If AChR antibodies are negative, muscle-specific kinase and lipoprotein-related 4 (LRP4) antibodies can also be obtained. Voltage-gated calcium channel antibodies can assist with diagnosis of LEMS. An ECG and troponin should be obtained to screen for myocarditis, and, if positive, a cardiology consultation and additional cardiac testing is advised. If myositis is suspected, liver enzymes, rheumatologic serologies, and a myositis antibody panel (including anti-HMG-CoA, see Chapter 18) should be tested.

Electrodiagnostic studies are recommended in these cases, including nerve conduction study (NCS) and electromyography (EMG) to evaluate for neuropathy or myopathy, as well as including neuromuscular junction testing with repetitive stimulation or single-fiber EMG. These studies are important because AChR antibodies can be nonspecific, and the absence of antibodies associated with myasthenia gravis does not exclude myasthenia gravis. Due to the indiscriminate nature of irAEs, electrodiagnostic studies can also help tease out if there are multiple overlapping processes (e.g., coexisting myasthenia gravis and myositis). MRI with and without contrast of the brain and/or spine can be considered depending on clinical suspicion and exam.

The management of ICPi-associated myasthenia gravis is guided by symptom severity and may include holding/discontinuing ICPi and starting corticosteroids. High-dose steroids may worsen symptoms in those with myasthenia gravis, and it is not known if this is also true for ICPi-associated myasthenia gravis, so caution is recommended. IVIg or plasma exchange should be started in patients with an incomplete response to steroids or with severe symptoms. It is not known if immunomodulatory therapies also counteract the treatment on the cancer itself. ICPi-associated myasthenia gravis may be monophasic and so long-term use of a steroid-sparing immunosuppressant may not be warranted.

In addition, pyridostigmine 30 mg orally three times a day can be trialed, with up-titration to 120 mg orally four times day. Rehab services, such as speech, occupational, and physical therapy should be engaged, and swallowing function should be assessed. Medications that can worsen myasthenia gravis, such as beta-blockers and aminoglycosides, should be avoided.

KEY POINTS TO REMEMBER

- Immune checkpoint inhibitors can cause a variety of neurologic immune-related adverse events that affect the central and peripheral nervous systems.
- Immune-related adverse events may overlap with each other (e.g., concurrent myasthenia gravis and myositis).
- The timing of immune-related adverse events can be idiosyncratic with administration of the drug.

Further Reading

Brahmer JR, Lacchetti C, Thompson JA. Management of immune-related adverse events in patients treated with immune checkpoint inhibitor therapy: American Society of Clinical Oncology Clinical Practice Guideline summary. *J Oncol Pract*. 2018;14(4):247–249.

Guidon AC. Lambert-Eaton Myasthenic syndrome, botulism, and immune checkpoint inhibitor-related myasthenia gravis. *Continuum (Minneap Minn)*. 2019;25(6):1785–1806.

Wang DY, Salem JE, Cohen JV, et al. Fatal toxic effects associated with immune checkpoint inhibitors: a systematic review and meta-analysis. *JAMA Oncol*. 2018;4(12):1721–1728.

14 Cauda Equina Syndrome

A 55-year-old man with a history of hypertension presents to the ED with acute lower back pain after falling from the top of a ladder while attaching Halloween decorations to his home. He denies head trauma or loss of consciousness. He could walk following the injury but experienced severe pain shooting down his right buttock. On arrival, his blood pressure is 130/70, his heart rate is 90, and he is afebrile. His neurologic exam shows intact mental status and cranial nerves and normal strength in the arms and legs except for the right leg, where effort is limited by pain. Both of you are surprised when you perform your sensory examination as he lacks sensation in the perianal area; his rectal tone is also low. Concerned, you obtain a bladder scan that shows 500 mL of retained urine after he attempts to void. An MRI reveals lumbar disc compression on the cauda equina.

What do you do now?

The possibility of cauda equina syndrome strikes fear into many practitioners, often because of its variable presentation as well as the need for urgent neuroimaging and treatment. The cauda equina, from the Latin "horse's tail," is the collection of nerve roots that includes L2 through L5, S1 through S5, and the coccygeal nerves. These nerve roots serve a variety of functions including lower extremity strength (L2 through S2) and sensation (L2 through S3), and perineal (S2 through S4) and coccygeal sensation (S4 through S5, coccygeal). Sacral portions of the cauda equina also mediate bladder function and external anal sphincter control. The most caudal end of the spinal cord is a cone-shaped region named the *conus medullaris*, which most commonly terminates at the L1–L2 disc level.

Due to their proximity, it is not always possible to differentiate a conus medullaris lesion from a process affecting the cauda equina. Conus medullaris lesions are more likely to have early bowel, bladder, and sexual dysfunction, which tend to be less pronounced in cauda equina lesions, as well as nonradicular back pain as opposed to radicular pain. Conus medullaris lesions are more likely to result in mild but symmetric leg weakness, whereas cauda equina lesions are more likely to result in asymmetric leg weakness, as seen with nerve root involvement. However, weakness may not be present in cauda equina syndrome—for example, in the setting of a central disc herniation that affects lower sacral or coccygeal nerve roots—so do not be falsely reassured if weakness is absent. Regardless, the presence of these symptoms warrants an urgent investigation, as discussed here.

Similarly, it can be challenging to differentiate cauda equina syndrome from a myelopathy or polyradiculoneuropathy. Features that may point toward cauda equina syndrome include a normal neurologic exam of the arms, absence of a cervical or thoracic sensory level, proximal leg weakness, reduced sensation in the legs or perineal region ("saddle anesthesia"), or reduced reflexes in the lower limbs. Reflexes include the patellar, Achilles tendon, anal wink, and bulbocavernosus reflexes. Early bladder impairment is often characterized by urinary retention, which may later become overflow incontinence. While often not elicited, it is also important to ask about the presence of sexual dysfunction, which can also be seen with cauda equina syndrome.

The causes of cauda equina syndrome are often divided into discogenic and nondiscogenic categories, but it can be helpful to instead think of

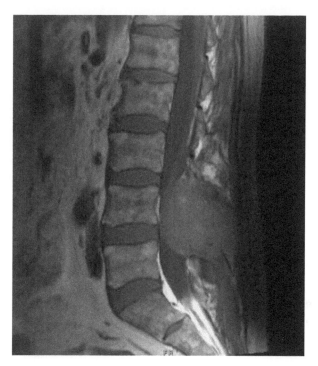

FIGURE 14.1 MRI of the lumbar spine showing a large, expansile destructive mass at approximately L4 resulting in severe canal stenosis and obliteration of the CSF space within the thecal sac.

compressive and noncompressive causes. These can be quickly delineated by the presence of a compression on MRI of the lumbosacral spine with and without contrast (see Figures 14.1 and 14.2). Compression may be caused by vertebral disc disease including disc herniation, vertebral body collapse, trauma, tumor, or focal infection, such as an epidural abscess. Intervertebral disc herniation is the most common cause of cauda equina syndrome. The most common tumors that affect the cauda equina are metastases, nerve sheath tumors, and ependymomas. Additional masses include epidural lipomatosis and epidural hematomas. Neoplastic or infectious infiltration of the vertebral bodies may lead to instability and compression.

While less common, noncompressive causes of cauda equina syndrome include inflammatory/autoimmune, infectious, and neoplastic processes. Acute inflammatory demyelinating polyneuropathy may cause

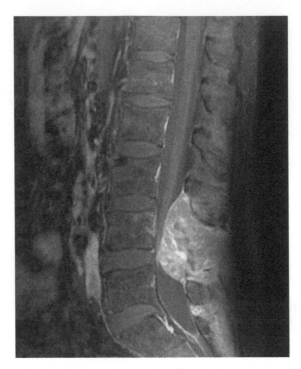

FIGURE 14.2 MRI of same lumbar spine mass, but with avid enhancement.

inflammation of the cauda equina, as can sarcoidosis, which can be visualized as nerve root enhancement on MRI with contrast. Inflammation of the arachnoid—arachnoiditis—may also present as cauda equina syndrome. Many infections can affect the cauda equina, especially viruses such as the herpes viruses (herpes simplex virus, varicella zoster virus, Epstein-Barr virus, and human cytomegalovirus), and bacterial infections, including Lyme disease and tuberculosis. Leptomeningeal metastases (carcinomatous meningitis) may also affect the cauda equina nerve roots.

Once cauda equina syndrome is suspected, urgent neuroimaging should be obtained. Plain radiographs may show a fracture, but ultimately an MRI is required to guide management. If an MRI cannot be obtained, then a CT myelogram should be considered. Compressive cauda equina syndrome requires urgent surgical management, especially in patients with a rapid onset of symptoms. If a noncompressive cause is suspected, electromyography can confirm this localization, though this may be falsely negative acutely. An LP looking for infectious and neoplastic etiologies will be helpful. Systemic imaging, including a PET, may also be helpful in order to identify additional areas of infection or neoplasm. Treatment of noncompressive cauda equina syndrome is specific to the underlying cause,

---

KEY POINTS TO REMEMBER

- Identifying cauda equina syndrome can be challenging, so maintain a high level of suspicion for this neurologic emergency.
- Symptoms can include sciatica, urinary/bowel impairment, back pain (with or without radicular symptoms), perineal anesthesia, and impaired sexual function.
- Urgent neuroimaging is crucial, preferably with MRI.
- Urgent consultation for surgical decompression should be sought in these cases.

Further Reading

Bennett SJ, Katzman GL, Roos RP, Mehta AS, Ali S. Neoplastic cauda equina syndrome: a neuroimaging-based review. *Pract Neurol.* 2016;16(1):35–41.

Lavy C, James A, Wilson-MacDonald J, Fairbank J. Cauda equina syndrome. *BMJ.* 2009;338:b936.

Todd NV, Dickson RA. Standards of care in cauda equina syndrome. *Br J Neurosurg.* 2016;30(5):518–522.

15 Intracranial Mass in a Person with HIV

A 40-year-old woman with a history of AIDS not on antiretrovirals (ARVs) (CD4 45, viral load >300,000) presented to the ED for generalized weakness, including progressive leg weakness over several weeks, headache, and confusion. She does not smoke tobacco or drink alcohol. General exam is notable for being ill-appearing, normotensive, and afebrile. Mental status exam is notable for somnolence but arouses briefly to voice, is oriented to hospital and city, and is able to follow one-step commands but falls asleep between them, requiring prompting. The remainder of the neurological exam is notable for right arm drift and symmetric 2+ reflexes; otherwise, her exam is limited by her mental status. A head CT reveals multifocal hypodense areas which are clearly enhancing on MRI.

What do you do now?

The differential diagnosis of a focal mass (either single or several) differs for patients with normal immune function and those with a compromised immune system, as in this patient. In patients who are immunocompetent, the differential includes infection, such as bacterial or parasitic causes like cysticercosis if there is a history of living in or travel to an endemic area, autoimmune disorders (e.g., multiple sclerosis, sarcoid), or neoplastic causes (primary or metastatic). In patients with HIV or AIDS, those on chemotherapy, transplant patients, or those immunosuppressed from other causes, the list should also include fungal abscess (like *Cryptococcus*), lymphoma, *Mycobacterium tuberculosis* (TB), *Toxoplasma gondii*, and *Nocardia* (see Box 15.1). Progressive multifocal leukoencephalopathy (PML) may also take the form of an apparent mass lesion in these patients. Clinical presentation does not help narrow the list very much, as most can present with headache, focal findings, and either seizures or depression of consciousness. Geographic location or exposure to foreign location may also be informative.

The CD4 count can guide the differential in patients with HIV. If the CD4 count is greater than 500/µL, the list of causes will be similar to immunocompetent patients. In patients with a CD4 count from 200 to 500/µL, focal brain lesions are less common than neuromuscular disorders (acute inflammatory demyelinating polyneuropathy, mononeuritis multiplex, peripheral neuropathy). A person meets criteria for AIDS with a CD4 count of less than 200/µL, which is when opportunistic infections (OIs) become most likely, including *Toxoplasma gondii, Cryptococcus,* and PML.

Imaging characteristics can be very helpful. The initial scan for a patient in the ED is likely going to be a head CT. This is especially important if

---

BOX 15.1 **Susceptibility for neurological disease based on CD4 count**

CD4 <400: Mononeuritis multiplex, Guillain-Barré syndrome, autoimmune conditions, peripheral neuropathy, syphilis
CD4 <200: *Toxoplasma gondii, Cryptococcus*, progressive multifocal leukoencephalopathy (PML), IRIS if recently started ARVs
CD4 <100: Primary CNS lymphoma, CMV, CNS TB, and all of the above

---

a lumbar puncture (LP) is planned in order to assess for herniation risk. Remember, head CT must be done before LP if the patient is immuno-compromised, older than 60 years, comatose, altered or with focal deficits, has a history of CNS disease, is presenting with a new seizure, or there is another reason to suspect a mass. Opening pressure measurement can be very helpful because an elevated opening pressure may point toward fungal infection (e.g., *Cryptococcus*). If the patient is known to have HIV, it is helpful to obtain the head CT with and without contrast to assess for enhancement. The head CT can also reveal calcification, which may be present in neurocysticercosis infection. However, MRI with and without contrast tends to be the most helpful, especially if a brain biopsy is ulti-mately warranted.

Intracranial lesions can be categorized by whether they are focal or diffuse, with or without mass effect (see Boxes 15.2 and 15.3). Focal lesions with mass effect include cerebral toxoplasmosis and primary CNS lymphoma, which can be challenging to distinguish on imaging alone. Cerebral toxo-plasmosis tends to result in multiple lesions, especially in the basal ganglia or gray–white junction, with ring or nodular enhancement and necrosis in the center, where as CNS lymphoma is more likely to be a single lesion with solid enhancement and restricted diffusion on diffusion-weighted imaging (DWI). Brain abscesses are thick-walled, with wall enhancement and significant edema. PML tends to be a focal lesion without mass effect, with abnormalities in the white matter extending to subcortical U fibers; these very rarely enhance, whereas cerebral tuberculoma may appear as variably enhancing small nodules without edema. Recent steroid use may eliminate any contrast enhancement and so imaging should be interpreted with this in mind.

But these characteristics are often not specific enough to help the ED physician or neurologist map out a definitive course for diagnosis and treatment. What are the best steps here? Large lesions with mass effect threatening herniation should signal the need for open biopsy with decompression. If this is not the case, the diagnosis may be made with serologic or CSF testing or systemic imaging, before pursuing biopsy. In addition to sending serologies and cultures, metagenomic next-generation sequencing and universal polymerase chain reaction (PCR) should be sent, especially if an infectious pathogen remains elusive. A detailed ophthalmology assessment can also be high yielding as it may show lymphoma, ocular toxoplasmosis, or CMV retinitis.

For CNS toxoplasmosis, serum *Toxoplasma* IgG is often positive, although it can be falsely negative. Consistent brain imaging and positive *Toxoplasma* IgG has a 90% predictive value for CNS toxoplasmosis, and so empiric treatment should be considered in those cases (see Figures 15.1 and 15.2). CNS *Cryptococcus* can be diagnosed with serum cryptococcal antigen (CrAg), which is very sensitive and specific in immunocompromised patients (but not adequate if immunocompromised). If PML is suspected, a positive CSF JC virus PCR can confirm the diagnosis. However, given variable sensitivity of this test, a negative CSF JC virus PCR despite clinical suspicion warrants brain biopsy for definitive diagnosis. Positive CSF Epstein-Barr virus (EBV) PCR may point toward primary CNS lymphoma. CSF cytology and flow cytometry can be helpful with diagnosis of lymphoma, but for increased sensitivity three separate LPs are recommended. The risks of LP in a patient with intracranial masses are significant, however, and CSF samples in many of the infectious processes may yield only

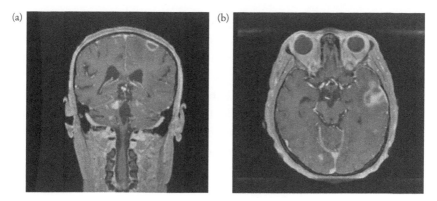

FIGURE 15.1 MRI of the brain with innumerable peripherally enhancing lesions in the supratentorial and infratentorial brain, some with vasogenic edema.

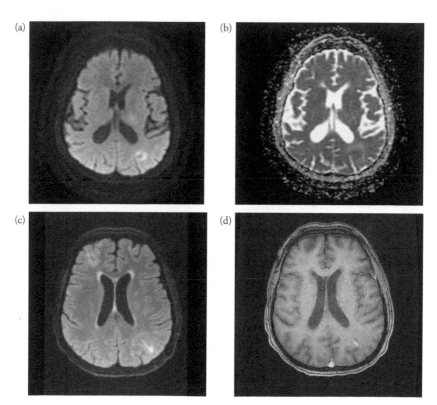

FIGURE 15.2 MRI of the brain with interval decrease in size and number of enhancing lesions as seen on DWI (a), ADC (b), T2 FLAIR (c), and gadolinium enhanced (d).

nonspecific pleocytosis and increased CSF protein. However, metagenomic sequencing and universal PCR may increase the yield. Blood cultures for bacteria and fungus and a search for an infectious source in the sinuses, ears, mouth and teeth, and heart should be done.

Systemic imaging may reveal other affected areas that can provide clues. Chest radiography can help to exclude tuberculosis, and, especially in smokers, it may reveal lung neoplasms. Concomitant pulmonary infection in an immunocompromised patient also raises concern for nocardiosis as a cause for brain abscess, which is treated with trimethoprim-sulfamethoxazole and can be missed with typical empiric antibiotics. PET CT may reveal more accessible lesions that are amenable to biopsy and should be considered before pursuing brain biopsy. PET and single positron emission CT (SPECT) can help to distinguish CNS lymphoma from other causes, as lymphoma tends to reveal hypermetabolic features whereas infections, including PML, are relatively hypometabolic.

If initial blood, spinal fluid, and imaging does not narrow a diagnosis, and whole-body PET is negative, stereotactic brain biopsy can be considered if the lesion is in a reasonable location. Areas of enhancement should be prioritized when deciding on a biopsy target. Empiric treatment of an infectious cause, such as toxoplasmosis, should result in a repeat MRI 2 weeks later to assess for improvement. Empiric steroid therapy might be tempting, and while it may improve symptoms or make the MRI look better, this does not help diagnosis and may delay definitive treatment if the lesion is primary CNS lymphoma—its use should be discouraged.

No algorithm is perfect, so clinical judgment and discussion with patients is crucial. And finally, of course, this patient needs to be treated for HIV infection with antiretrovirals—watching closely for the development of immune reconstitution inflammatory syndrome (IRIS)—and have her leukocyte counts and general health closely monitored.

- An updated CD4 count can help narrow the differential.
- In addition to sending serologies and cultures, metagenomic next-generation sequencing and universal PCR should be sent, especially if concerned for an infectious pathogen.
- Toxoplasmosis is a common infectious cause of intracranial mass lesions; however, a number of other infectious, neoplastic, and other processes may present in this way.
- Neuroimaging, especially MRI with contrast, can help to distinguish between some of these conditions.
- If the diagnosis is elusive, biopsy is recommended. Sometimes an alternate biopsy target can be found on whole-body PET CT before pursuing brain biopsy.

Further Reading

American Academy of Neurology Quality Standards Committee. Evaluation and management of intracranial mass lesions in AIDS. *Neurology.* 1998;50:21–26.

Antinori A, Ammassari A, De Luca A, et al. Diagnosis of AIDS-related focal brain lesions: a decision-making analysis based on clinical and neuroradiologic characteristics combined with polymerase chain reaction assays in CSF. *Neurology.* 1997;48:687–694.

Antinori A, Ammassari A, Luzzati R, et al. Role of brain biopsy in the management of focal brain lesions in HIV-infected patients. Gruppo Italiano Cooperativo AIDS & Tumori. *Neurology.* 2000;54:993.

Marra CM. Central nervous system infection with *Toxoplasma gondii.* Handb Clin Neurol. 2018;152:117–122.

Stenzel W, Pels H, Staib P, et al. Concomitant manifestation of primary CNS lymphoma and *Toxoplasma* encephalitis in a patient with AIDS. *J Neurol.* 2004;251:764.

16 Rapidly Progressive Dementia

You are asked to consult on a 46-year-old woman on the inpatient psychiatric service to "rule out frontotemporal dementia." For the past several months she has been "acting strangely," seeming depressed, anhedonic, and apathetic. She is single, having lived alone for 12 years after a difficult divorce. Medical history includes chronic depression and migraine headaches. Current medications include citalopram and clonazepam, which seemed to improve her mood and behavior. However, over the past several days, she has worsened and is distinctly less involved with her care team who are diagnosing a form of catatonic psychosis. Vital signs have been stable. She is afebrile. Neck is supple, and general exams have been normal. She tends to assume a fetal position but relaxes intermittently with good limb movements, and she is able to answer some questions. Facial movements are symmetric, motor tone is diffusely increased, and reflexes are brisk with Babinski signs bilaterally.

What do you do now?

This alarming case seems psychiatric but is unexpectedly not responding at all to medications. That has appropriately raised red flags to the psychiatry team. In addition, the hyperreflexia and dyskinetic movements are suggestive of neurological disease. History here is so sparse that it is important not to make too many assumptions about the timing of her symptomatology: it could be chronic or subacute, and things seemingly are worsening. The search for treatable neurological disease is paramount, and the best next intervention would be to obtain head imaging, followed by a lumbar puncture. Following this, an EEG would be ideal not only to investigate the possibility of seizures, but also to search for clues of focal or generalized cortical or subcortical dysfunction (Box 16.1).

Possibilities here include rapid dementia and relatively slow encephalitis or encephalopathy. This patient's presentation is reminiscent of frontotemporal dementia (FTD), in particular the semantic variant primary progressive aphasia form. However, the course here seems much more

---

BOX 16.1   **Differential diagnosis in subacute encephalopathy**

Multi-infarct dementia
Primary CNS angiopathy
Cerebral amyloid angiopathy
Lyme disease
HIV dementia
Neurosyphilis
Whipple's disease
Wernicke encephalopathy
Vitamin B12 deficiency
Hepatic encephalopathy
Porphyria
Autoimmune encephalitis (paraneoplastic encephalitis; limbic
    encephalitis)
Medication effects
Creuzfeld-Jacob disease
Frontotemporal dementia
Lewy body dementia

rapidly progressive than FTD, although a fuller history could, of course, provide clues to a longer progression.

The motor changes and subacute presentation can suggest encephalitis, though not typical of common viral encephalitides like herpes simplex or zoster encephalitis (or Eastern and Western Equine, West Nile, and other less common encephalitides), which are much more rapidly progressive and manifest with early headache and altered consciousness and cognition. Also, MRI typically will show parenchymal abnormalities once the course of the disease has progressed. Herpes zoster encephalitis can sometimes progress more slowly. For example, there are a number of reports of this more subacute presentation in patients with AIDS. Metabolic encephalopathies seem unlikely here with normal lab values. Syphilitic meningoencephalitis is possible, even though risk factors are not apparent and VDRL was normal. Lyme disease, ehrlichiosis, and cat-scratch fever are also said to sometimes cause a slowly progressive encephalopathy, but the prominent behavioral features in our case with a paucity of exam findings suggest an autoimmune encephalitis (AE).

Anti-NMDA-receptor encephalitis is an often paraneoplastic autoimmune attack on NMDA receptors in the brain, generally affects younger patients, and initially presents with altered behavior, progressing to worsening mental status, catatonia, and focal neurological deficits including aphasia, weakness, ataxia, and eventually seizures and coma. High rates of co-occurring tumors, particularly teratomas that contain NMDA receptors, suggest that an autoimmune response develops. But no tumors are ever found in many patients. MRI can be normal, as are routine labs and inflammatory markers such as ESR and CRP. EEG can reveal slowing and epileptiform discharges. CSF usually reveals lymphocytic pleocytosis, elevated protein with normal glucose, elevated IgG index, and unique oligoclonal bands. Diagnosis can be made with identification of NMDAR antibody in serum or CSF, and often it is tested in both specimens. In female-bodied individuals, it is important to search for an ovarian teratoma with use of ultrasound or MRI and to rescreen if initially negative (Table 16.1).

AMPA receptor encephalitis seems also to usually result from paraneoplastic autoimmune activity, and, like NMDAR encephalitis, most patients will ultimately be found to have a solid organ tumor. Clinical

TABLE 16.1 **Tumors associated with autoimmune encephalopathy**

NMDA receptor	Ovarian or mediastinal teratoma
AMPA receptor	Lung, breast cancer, thymoma
Hu	Small cell lung cancer (SCLC), neuroendocrine tumors
Yo	Ovarian cancer, breast cancer
CV2/CRMP5	SCLC, thymoma
Ri	SCLC, breast cancer, gynecologic cancer
Ma2	Testicular, breast, lung, stomach cancer
Amphiphysin	SCLC, breast cancer
Recoverin	SCLC, Non-SCLC
LGI1	Thymoma, thyroid cancer, lung cancer, renal cell cancer
Caspr2	Thymoma
GABA B receptor	SCLC
GABA A receptor	Thymoma, Hodgkin's lymphoma, multiple myeloma
MGluR5	Hodgkin's lymphoma
DPPX	Unknown
Glycine receptor	Thymoma, lymphoma, breast cancer

symptoms share characteristics with NMDAR encephalitis, with altered behavior and thinking initially (which usually leads to psychiatric evaluation) followed by focal neurologic deficits such as aphasia, paresis, ataxia, and later catatonia, seizures, and coma. Hyperreflexia, Babinski reflexes, and posturing are often seen.

Management of AE relies on early diagnosis and immunomodulation as soon as infectious etiologies are ruled out. Antibody screening is wise as is polymerase chain reaction (PCR) testing for all possible infectious agents including herpes simplex and zoster. A search for a tumor which might be the etiologic source is essential, as resection and treatment can lead to recovery with no other intervention.

A number of interventions for the management of AE have been promoted including corticosteroids, plasma exchange, IVIg, rituximab, and cyclophosphamide. Currently there is not a consensus on which should be employed first or the duration of therapy. Prognosis is generally good if treatment is begun relatively soon after the disease becomes apparent. Our presenting case has progressed, and the ultimate outcome is not clear. Even when treatment is successful, relapses can occur, sometimes months or years later.

KEY POINTS TO REMEMBER

· AEs often present with psychiatric symptoms, although they may progress to more overt neurological presentations including focal seizures, paresis, and depressed consciousness.
· Lab testing and imaging can be normal in AEs, and CSF analysis is essential to rule out treatable infectious encephalitis and to confirm the immunological etiology.
· Specific treatment of AE is debatable, but plasma exchange, IVIG, or immune modulators are the mainstay of treatment, with relative good prognosis possible with reasonably early treatment.

Further Reading

Budhram A, Silverman M, Burneo JG. Neurosyphilis mimicking autoimmune encephalitis in a 52-year-old man. *CMAJ*. 2017;189(29):E962–E965.
Dalmau J, Armangué T, Planagumà J, et al. An update on anti-NMDA receptor encephalitis for neurologists and psychiatrists: mechanisms and models. *Lancet Neurol*. 2019;18:1045–1057.
Olney NT, Spina S, Miller BL. Frontotemporal dementia. *Neurol Clin*. 2017;35(2):339–374.

17 Functional Hemiparesis

A 45-year-old man began noticing weakness on his right side 2 days ago, gradually worsening. He denies previous symptoms of weakness and has had no recent trauma. General exam is normal. A screening mental status exam is normal. Cranial nerves all seem to be normal except for numbness to touch on the right side of his face, normalizing at the midline. He has "give-way weakness" in all muscles of the right arm and leg. Hoover's sign is positive (lack of left hip extensor muscle activity when asked lift his right leg). Muscle tone is normal, reflexes are all in the 2+ range, and there are no abnormal motor movements. Gait fluctuates; you note dramatic wavering and near falling when supporting some weight on the right leg. Sensation to touch and temperature is reduced in the right arm and leg, and there is numbness on the right side of his trunk normalizing at the midline. CT scan of the head is normal. Basic labs are also normal.

What do you do now?

BOX 17.1   **Conversion disorder (functional neurological symptom disorder)**

Diagnostic criteria

A. One or more symptoms of altered voluntary motor or sensory function
B. Clinical findings provide evidence of incompatibility between the symptom and recognized neurological or medical conditions
C. The symptom or deficit is not better explained by another medical or mental disorder
D. The symptom of deficit causes clinically significant distress or impairment in social, occupational, or other important areas of functioning or warrants medical evaluation

From American Psychiatric Association, *Diagnostic and Statistical Manual of Mental Disorders* (5th ed.).

This patient seems to be suffering from a conversion disorder (CD; a functional neurological symptom disorder), now classified as one of the somatic symptoms and related disorders in the *Diagnostic and Statistical Manual of Mental Disorders of the American Psychiatric Association, Fifth Edition* (*DSM-5*) (Box 17.1). This group of disorders was formerly known as *somatoform disorders* and are also known as *functional disorders*, implying normal neurological function with overlying disability of unknown cause, presumably psychogenic. CD has been explained in different ways but is generally presumed to be the result of significant unresolved psychological factors, particularly trauma, and can be viewed as adaptive. Symptoms of CD commonly include weakness/paralysis, involuntary movements, sensory losses, ataxia, visual dysfunction, nonepileptic seizures (psychogenic nonepileptic spells [PNES]), and other alterations in consciousness (see Box 17.2).

Diagnosis of CD must be made carefully in order to avoid missing neurological disease. A careful exam with clear documentation is essential as multiple exams over time can be decisive. While many features of the neurological exam depend on reliable patient cooperation, there are some

Weakness does not follow corticospinal, myotomal, or peripheral
  nerve pattern
Normal reflexes, tone, and posture with paralysis
Variable resistance over time
Variable resistance against variable force
Give-way weakness, especially against very light force
Drift without pronation
Observe inadvertent movements awake (perhaps with distraction)
  and asleep
Hoover's sign in someone with asymmetric weakness
Reverse hands/fingers with strength testing
Vibration and other sensation loss splitting the midline
Nonanatomic distribution of sensory loss
Astasia abasia

elements that can objectively provide evidence for CD. In cases of motor
dysfunction, suggestive clues for CD include the presence of "give-way"
weakness (initial full-power on manual testing, followed by relaxation),
fluctuation in power over a short period of time, inconsistency of strength
testing when done in different ways (such as our patient with plantarflexion),
and patterns of weakness that cannot be explained anatomically. Normal
reflexes and lack of abnormal postures or tone differences are all clues as
well. On exam of pronator drift, falling of the arm without pronation can
be seen. Another clue to non-neurological paralysis is "Hoover's sign," a lack
of contralateral hip extension (by the otherwise strong leg) to support the
"weak" hip flexion; however, this is only helpful with unilateral weakness as
hip extension must be possible with the contralateral, strong leg. Moving
of the paralyzed limb during sleep, if observed, constitutes good evidence
of CD. Another good way to induce movement in the weak limb is to have
the patient cross fingers or hands and rapidly ask for right and left actions.
Clues to functional sensory loss include nonanatomical presentations such
as facial numbness including the angle of the jaw (C2) in otherwise trigeminal region of facial numbness; facial numbness stopping at the hairline (V1

extends to vertex); sensory loss stopping at wrist, elbow, shoulder, knee, or groin; and "midline-splitting" sensory loss, as in our patient. Vision loss can be circumvented by asking the patient to do something that requires good vision or watching them do very poorly at something (like fingertip touching) that requires proprioception but not vision. Functional movement disorders such as tremors or more dramatic dyskinetic movements tend to vary with situation and with suggestibility and distraction. Unusual gaits appearing extremely unstable but without falling ("astasia-abasia") can be seen. Mental status is not particularly telling in CD, and in particular, the famous *la belle indifference* (unconcerned demeanor) is overrated as a diagnostic feature of CD.

Managing functional neurological illness is challenging even when other neurological conditions have been reliably ruled out. It is important to remember that the symptoms manifested by patients with CD are quite real to them and a source of distress and disability. Many treatment approaches have been promoted, including cognitive therapy, physical therapy, and psychoactive medications. Most would now agree that a direct confrontational approach in the acute setting is generally not fruitful. Rather, a compassionate, non-judgmental discussion of higher-level brain "software" problems as causal in the condition will set the stage for gradual improvement with physical and psychotherapeutic interventions. As patients with CD may have underlying psychiatric illness, asking about suicidal ideation is important.

A related disorder, also in the DSM-5's Somatic Symptom chapter, is *factitious disorder,* which consists of "falsification" of signs and symptoms with the purpose of deception. Unlike CD, the patient is well aware of the pretense. It is distinguished from malingering (though closer than to CD) in that the benefit to the patient is more obscure. A typical example is the patient with a functional neurological presentation for whom the "sick role" is beneficial on a social/psychological level but without clear gain (such as financial gains or freedom from prosecution). These distinctions are often complex, but important, as approaches to CD, factitious disorder, and malingering will be different.

Another related disorder, *somatic symptom disorder,* is generally not a presenting factor in emergency settings but can certainly complicate neurological presentations in the ED. This condition is characterized by multiple concurrent distressing symptoms including pain, nausea, dizziness, and fatigue. There are often underlying medical illnesses which serve to heighten the patient's vigilance and awareness of somatic complaints. The patient tends to be highly anxious and worried about their symptoms as compared with patients with CD, and they are often very resistant to approaches consisting of reassurance.

KEY POINTS TO REMEMBER

- CD (functional neurological symptom disorder) simulates neurological disease but can generally be distinguished with careful observation, neurological exam, and testing.
- Typical presentations of CD include motor weakness, movement abnormalities, ataxia, sensory changes, alterations in consciousness, and spells concerning for seizure.
- Management of CD centers around appropriate testing and sharing reassuring normal test results with the patient, followed by a plan for treatment, often involving cognitive and behavioral techniques, with predicted gradual improvement and even resolution of symptoms.
- Factitious disorder and malingering are distinguished from CD by the patient's conscious effort to deceive.

Further Reading

American Psychiatric Association. Somatic symptom and related disorders. In *Diagnostic and statistical manual of mental disorders (DSM-5)*. Washington, DC: American Psychiatric Association Publishing; 2013: 309–327.

Daum C, Hubschmid M, Aybek S. The value of "positive" clinical signs for weakness, sensory and gait disorders in conversion disorder: a systematic and narrative review. *J Neurol Neurosurg Psychiatry*. 2014;85(2):180–190.

Richardson M, Isbister G, Nicholson B. A novel treatment protocol (nocebo hypothesis cognitive behavioural therapy; NH-CBT) for functional neurological symptom disorder/conversion disorder: a retrospective consecutive case series. *Behav Cogn Psychother*. 2018;46(4):497–503.

Stone J, Edwards M. Trick or treat? Showing patients with functional (psychogenic) motor symptoms their physical signs. *Neurology*. 2012;79(3):282–284.

18 Acute Myopathy

A 70-year-old man with diabetes and hyperlipidemia presents with difficulty swallowing. Two weeks ago, he noticed leg weakness, and then arm weakness, especially in his deltoids. One week ago, he developed double vision; 4 days ago, he choked when drinking liquids. Vital signs show a heart rate 104, blood pressure 142/80, and oxygen saturation 97% on room air. Exam is notable for normal mental status; speaking in full sentences; with reactive pupils; full extraocular muscles; and bifacial, tongue, and neck flexion weakness, as well as weakness in his proximal arms and legs. There are no muscle fasciculations. Sensation is intact. Reflexes are present except at the ankles. Labs include normal chemistries and CBC, mild transaminitis, creatine kinase (CK) 4,500, and negative troponin. He has no family history of a neuromuscular disease.

What do you do now?

Before considering the localization for these symptoms, it is important to recognize potential life-threatening clues on this exam. Neck flexion weakness is a good surrogate for diaphragmatic weakness and should raise concern for respiratory insufficiency. For this reason, bedside respiratory function tests are recommended. It is especially helpful to ask respiratory therapy to measure the functional vital capacity (FVC) and maximal inspiratory force (MIF). One can anticipate need for intubation for FVC <15–20 cc/kg (or <1 liter), MIF ≤25 cm H_2O (where approximately –50 cm H_2O is normal), or for rapid worsening. In the acute period, MIF and FVC can be measured multiple times a day to assess for crucial changes. While less precise, respiratory capacity can also be assessed and trended by asking the patient to count out loud as quickly as possible using one breath (normal is approximately 40). Importantly, while these patients should have pulse oximetry monitoring because oxygen saturation can be falsely reassuring. In neuromuscular respiratory weakness, hypercarbia often occurs before hypoxemia, and so once the pulse oximeter starts beeping, your patient is already in crisis.

What might cause this patient's constellation of symptoms? The lack of upper motor neuron features makes brain or spinal cord involvement less likely. Normal sensation and overall intact reflexes make nerve root and nerve far less likely. There is no history of fluctuating weakness, but the bulbar symptoms and limb weakness may be consistent with a neuromuscular junction process. However, the most likely localization, given preserved sensation, muscle soreness, proximal muscle weakness, and elevated creatine kinase, is muscle (Box 18.1).

Myopathies can be caused by a multitude of factors, including medications, systemic disease (e.g., HIV), genetic disorders, and inflammatory diseases. If suspicious for a myopathy, the CK can help narrow the differential. Elevated CK may be found in toxic myopathies, inflammatory myopathies (synonym: myositis), and infection-related myopathies. A normal or low CK can be seen with endocrine myopathy (e.g., thyroid disease), critical illness myopathy, and some congenital myopathies. While inflammatory myopathies usually present with high CK, the CK may return to normal if partially treated, so inquiring about recent steroid use is crucial.

BOX 18.1 **Causes of myopathy**

Inflammatory
- Antisynthetase syndrome
- Dermatomyositis
- Immune-mediated necrotizing myopathy
- Inclusion body myositis
- Overlap syndromes: Lupus, Sjögren's syndrome, scleroderma
- Vasculitis

Noninflammatory
- Toxic: HMG-CoA reductase inhibitors, corticosteroids, alcohol
- Electrolyte: Hypokalemia, hypophosphatemia, hypocalcemia
- Infectious: Bacterial (e.g., Lyme), viral (e.g., HIV, CMV, EBV), fungal, parasitic (e.g., toxoplasmosis, trichinosis)
- Rhabdomyolysis: Seizure, crush/trauma, hyperthermia
- Inherited: Muscular dystrophy, acid maltase deficiency

The time course can also help narrow the differential. Rapidly progressive myopathies, especially with elevated CK, are more likely to be a toxic myopathy, such as due to a drug. One of the most important drug classes to consider are statins, which can cause a toxic myopathy, especially in older individuals and when used in combination with drugs that affect statin metabolism (e.g., cytochrome P450 inhibitors), or cause an immune-mediated necrotizing myopathy as described below. Other key drugs to ask about if considering a toxic myopathy are amiodarone, colchicine, corticosteroids, ethanol, fibrates, and zidovudine, though the list of possible drugs is extensive and so obtaining a full and accurate medication history (including supplements) is crucial. The treatment of a toxic myopathy is removal of the drug.

There is a growing recognition of immune-mediated myopathies. This class of myopathy can be distinguished from other types of myopathy based on biopsy characteristics. Biopsy can be helpful since an antibody cannot always be identified, and this type of myopathy is often treatable. The most common inflammatory myopathies are immune-mediated necrotizing myopathies, dermatomyositis, antisynthetase syndrome, and inclusion body myositis. These subtypes are associated with specific antibodies that are helpful to identify as they can predict the development of extramuscular disease, including dermatologic, cardiac, and pulmonary complications, and even malignancies.

Immune-mediated necrotizing myopathies feature severe, often acute proximal muscle weakness. The two main antibodies associated with this type of myopathy are anti-HMG-CoA and anti-SRP, though no antibody is identified in a large fraction of cases. In addition to a toxic myopathy, statins can cause an immune-mediated necrotizing myopathy due to the presence of an antibody against HMG-CoA reductase, though up to a third of patients with this antibody have no known statin exposure. The treatment of immune-mediated necrotizing myopathy is immunomodulatory therapy, including high-dose corticosteroids and often steroid-sparing immunosuppressive agents. There is rarely extramuscular involvement in immune-mediated necrotizing myopathy.

Dermatomyositis is often characterized by subacute proximal muscle weakness and rash. This rash is erythematous and involves photosensitive areas of the face including eyelids (heliotrope), shoulders, and extensor surfaces of the joints. In addition to skin, there can also be cardiac involvement resulting in cardiac arrhythmias, heart failure, or myocarditis, as well as the development of interstitial lung disease. Dermatomyositis is associated with malignancy.

Antisynthetase syndrome is associated with antibodies to aminoacyl transfer RNA synthetases and these are associated with an array of clinical features, including diseases of the heart and lungs. These patients can develop similar skin findings as in dermatomyositis. The presence of an anti-antisynthetase antibody with evidence of collagen disease (e.g., systemic lupus erythematosus) is also classified as an overlap myositis.

Inclusion body myositis is distinct in that it is slowly progressive and tends to affect the deep finger flexors and quadriceps. While the other inflammatory myopathies are generally responsive to immunotherapy, inclusion body myositis is not.

Consider sending a myositis panel to test for known antibodies associated with inflammatory myopathies prior to starting any immunomodulatory therapy because treatment can result in false negatives. Identification of an antibody can guide the need for searching for concomitant extramuscular disease. Of note, despite increasing recognition, most panels do not include anti-HMG-CoA and so this must be sent separately.

Nerve conduction study (NCS) and electromyography (EMG) can assist with confirming the diagnosis of myopathy and with identifying potential muscle targets for biopsy. A muscle biopsy is often more helpful when the CK is elevated than when it is normal.

In addition to identification and treatment of the myopathy, it is important to also remember the downstream complications of myopathy, like myoglobinuria resulting in acute kidney injury and deconditioning requiring assistance from rehabilitative services.

The patient described here was confirmed to have a myopathy on NCS/EMG. His statin was stopped on admission. He tested positive for anti-HMG-CoA. He received pulse steroids and intravenous immunoglobulin with excellent clinical response.

KEY POINTS TO REMEMBER

- Neck flexion strength is an important surrogate for respiratory muscle strength.
- Neuromuscular respiratory weakness causes hypercarbia before hypoxemia.
- Myopathies can be associated with high and normal/low creatinine kinase, which can help inform the differential.
- Toxic myopathy is the most common cause of acute myopathies that predominantly affect proximal muscles. A thorough review of recent medications, including supplements, is required.
- Inflammatory myopathy (myositis) can be associated with extramuscular diseases that can affect the skin, heart, and lungs, as well as be associated with malignancy.
- Statins can cause both a toxic myopathy and an immune-mediated necrotizing myopathy (anti-HMG-CoA).
- Consider sending a myositis antibody panel, as well as anti-HMG-CoA, before starting immunomodulatory therapy. Identification of an antibody can help guide workup of associated diseases and direct treatment.

Further Reading

Goyal NA. Immune-mediated myopathies. *Continuum (Minneap Minn).* 2019;25(6):1564–1585.

Schmidt J. Current classification and management of inflammatory myopathies. *J Neuromuscul Dis.* 2018;5(2):109–129.

Treatment Dilemmas

19 Cardioembolic Stroke with Contraindications to Anticoagulation

A 74-year-old man with chronic atrial fibrillation was directed to discontinue warfarin therapy 3 months ago when he was found to have significant iron deficiency anemia with blood in the stool but negative endoscopic and radiologic workup of his GI tract. Last week he had a transient left visual field loss, and this morning, about 8 hours prior to presenting to the ED, he noticed difficulty with speech after getting out of the shower. In the remote past he had a left cerebellar stroke which led to transient ataxia and vertigo, at which time the atrial fibrillation was discovered. Today, his heart rate is irregular at approximately 76 beats per minute, atrial fibrillation is identified on ECG, and blood pressure (BP) is 134/76 mm Hg. General exam is normal, but on neurological exam there is some difficulty with naming low-frequency objects, and fluency is reduced. Basic labs are normal, including coagulation studies. CT today reveals the old cerebellar stroke and a question of attenuation changes in the cortex near the left Sylvian fissure but is otherwise normal.

What do you do now?

This patient is likely having recurrent cerebral ischemic events, probably occurring due to cardiac thromboemboli. After confirming this, your next thought should be about ways to prevent further strokes. Anticoagulation is appropriate but there are understandable concerns. First is the fact that this patient was felt to be a risk for serious GI bleeding. The second is that there is likely to be a new area of infarction, which can undergo hemorrhagic conversion, which is more likely if the patient is anticoagulated. He is out of the window for tissue plasminogen activator (tPA). So it is time to assess the risk of anticoagulation versus the risk of a new cardioembolic event while keeping his unique risk factors for bleeding in mind.

First, let's tackle the GI bleeding issue. His blood count is normal and there is no active GI bleeding; his previous GI workup was negative. The ideal timing to restart anticoagulation remains poorly characterized. For patients with a high risk of ischemic stroke from atrial fibrillation estimated with a CHA2DS2-VASc Score and low risk of rebleeding, resumption of anticoagulation can be considered within a few days (Table 19.1). Patients with a higher risk of bleeding but lower risk of thromboembolism may benefit from a more delayed start. Hematocrit should be followed closely, and the patient should remain vigilant for evidence of rebleeding.

TABLE 19.1 **CHA2DS2-VASc score calculation**

Category	+0 Points	+1 Point	+2 Points
Age (years)	< 65	65–74	≥ 75
Sex	Male	Female	–
Congestive heart failure history	No	Yes	–
Hypertension history	No	Yes	–
Stroke/TIA/thromboembolism history	No	–	Yes
Vascular disease history	No	Yes	–
Diabetes history	No	Yes	–

Score 0: "low" risk, may not require anticoagulation
Score 1: "low-moderate" risk, consider antiplatelet or anticoagulation
Score 2: "moderate-high" risk, consider anticoagulation

What about the risk of converting an ischemic infarction into a hemorrhagic one? Evidence is controversial here, too. The size of the acute infarction is probably important (i.e., a large infarction is more likely to bleed). Avoiding very high spikes in BP and careful monitoring of coagulation studies will bias the odds against intracerebral hemorrhage. On the other hand, acutely lowering BP in acute stroke can lead to extension of the infarctions so the risk must be balanced. MRI can help estimate the size of the stroke and can also detect even small amounts of bleeding, which could inform anticoagulation decisions. But, back to the original question: Will the reduction in risk of recurrent infarction be outweighed by the risk of hemorrhagic conversion and resulting morbidity and mortality risks? It turns out that the risks tend to balance out pretty closely. Thus, evidence here is mixed.

Is there any advantage to using low-molecular weight heparin (LMWH)? No; in fact, there are disadvantages. The half-life of LMWH is long, and it is inactivated by protamine to a much lesser extent. Therefore, if there is a bleeding complication, heparin is easier to reverse. Also, its activity is not assessable by partial thromboplastin time (PTT), so the degree of anticoagulation is generally inferred. And it is expensive (Table 19.2).

So, what to do in terms of attempting to prevent recurrent cerebral ischemia in this patient? Since evidence does not really help, this becomes a clinical judgment problem. But, you are not alone. This patient and his family can and should be enlisted to weigh the pros and cons. What they need to know is that the next stroke can be devastating, but that it is impossible to know when or if this will happen. Echocardiography can help by ruling out an intracardiac thrombus, but of course this is just a snapshot, and thrombi can begin to form at any time. The chances of recurrent stroke happening are generally below 5% in the first several days, so odds are good that this will not occur while they are weighing the options acutely. MRI can help by delineating the size of the stroke. Perhaps it is small but with a penumbra of impending ischemia, therefore less likely to bleed than a large area of infarcted tissue. If the patient and family opt to avoid anticoagulation, this decision can be reassessed over the next few days. Cardiological consultation about acute and long-term plans for dealing with the atrial fibrillation with medication, cardioversion, or ablation therapy might help but the success rate of these interventions has not been high enough to obviate the need for anticoagulation.

TABLE 19.2 **Comparison of oral anticoagulants for stroke prophylaxis in patients with nonvalvular atrial fibrillation**

Anticoagulant	Warfarin	Apixaban (Eliquis)	Dabigatran (Pradaxa)	Rivaroxaban (Xarelto)
Mechanism	Vitamin K antagonist	Selective direct factor Xa inhibitor	Competitive direct thrombin inhibitor	Selective direct factor Xa inhibitor
Routine level monitoring	Variable: semi-weekly to monthly	None	None	None
Dosing frequency	Per pharmacist	Twice daily	Twice daily	Nightly
Dosing considera-tions	No renal dose adjustment.	Dose adjustment based on age, weight, and/or renal function	Dose adjustment based on renal function	Dose adjustment based on renal function
Antidote	10 mg vitamin K IV and four-factor prothrombin complex concentrate (if not available, use fresh frozen plasma).	Andexanet alfa (AndexXa)	Idarucizumab (Praxbind)	Andexanet alfa (AndexXa)
Comparison with warfarin for stroke prevention		ARISTOTLE: Superior to warfarin	RELY: Superior to warfarin in intention-to-treat analysis	ROCKET-AF: Non-inferior to warfarin.

KEY POINTS TO REMEMBER

- Both systemic bleeding and intracerebral bleeding risks must be considered before starting anticoagulation in the acute post-stroke setting.
- MRI of the brain and echocardiography can help the neurologist and patient weigh the risks and benefits of starting anticoagulation.

- Unless there is a contraindication, an antiplatelet should be started and then switched to anticoagulation when appropriate.
- If anticoagulation is begun in the acute post-stroke setting, strict control of BP and close monitoring of bleeding parameters is essential.

Further Reading

Connolly SJ, Ezekowitz MD, Yusuf S, et al. Dabigatran versus warfarin in patients with atrial fibrillation. *N Engl J Med.* Sep 17 2009;361(12):1139–1151.

Granger CB, Alexander JH, McMurray JJ, et al. Apixaban versus warfarin in patients with atrial fibrillation. *N Engl J Med.* Sep 15 2011;365(11):981–992.

Kernan WN, Ovbiagele B, Black HR, et al. Guidelines for the prevention of stroke in patients with stroke and transient ischemic attack: a guideline for healthcare professionals from the American Heart Association/American Stroke Association. *Stroke.* Jul 2014;45(7):2160–2236.

Paciaroni M, Agnelli G, Falocci N, et al. Early recurrence and cerebral bleeding in patients with acute ischemic stroke and atrial fibrillation: effect of anticoagulation and its timing: the RAF Study. *Stroke.* Aug 2015;46(8):2175–2182.

Patel MR, Mahaffey KW, Garg J, et al. Rivaroxaban versus warfarin in nonvalvular atrial fibrillation. *N Engl J Med.* Sep 8 2011;365(10):883–891.

Sacchetti DC, Furie KL, Yaghi S. Cardioembolic stroke: mechanisms and therapeutics. *Semin Neurol.* Jun 2017;37(3):326–338.

Witt DM, Delate T, Garcia DA, et al. Risk of thromboembolism, recurrent hemorrhage, and death after warfarin therapy interruption for gastrointestinal tract bleeding. *Arch Intern Med.* Oct 22 2012;172(19):1484–1491.

20 Recurring Transient Ischemic Attack

A 73-year-old man was noted by his wife to abruptly slur his speech and complain of right arm clumsiness earlier this evening, which resolved within minutes. These symptoms recurred several hours later, this time lasting for 10 minutes, before completely resolving again. He is now in the ED despite his unwillingness to have medical care and admits that symptoms like today's have bothered him in the past. He denies head pain, chest pain, and shortness of breath. Medical history is only remarkable for hypertension that has been well controlled. He has no other neurological history. His general exam is normal except for cataracts. His blood pressure (BP) is 128/67, heart rate is 78 and regular, and there are no cardiac murmurs. His neurological exam is normal. A noncontrast CT scan of the head shows some mild cortical atrophy but is otherwise unremarkable. He has made it clear that he intends to go home.

What do you do now?

This presentation is most likely to be the result of recurrent transient ischemia to the brain. The localization is probably the subcortical left frontal region since the arm and articulatory muscles seem most affected. For this reason, there is a suspicion of left middle cerebral artery (MCA) involvement. However, the lack of cognitive/dysphasic symptoms might suggest posterior circulation. Upper and lower limbs should be equally affected when pathological processes affect the corticospinal tract in the brainstem, but this rule is not entirely reliable. Could this presentation reflect nonischemic CNS dysfunction? Acephalgic migraine (migraine aura without headache) can occur in his age group, but very rarely in patients without a history of migraine. A seizure affecting the motor cortex can affect articulation and limb strength, so this is another possibility. However, migraine auras and focal seizures are generally manifested by "positive phenomena": in the case of migraine, by paresthesias, visual images, and scotomata; in the case of focal seizures, by dystonic or clonic activity rather than by weakness. It is possible that observers did not note a focal seizure, with subsequent Todd's paralysis mimicking the weakness of a transient ischemic attack (TIA). Another possibility is so-called recrudescence of symptoms from an old stroke on the basis of infectious, metabolic, or hypoperfusion conditions. In the presenting case, the CT does not reveal a prior stroke, and so this is less likely. The diagnosis of TIA is a clinical one. Given the risk of subsequent completed infarct, it is prudent to take such symptoms seriously.

If this patient's recurrent symptoms do indeed stem from focal ischemia, what are the possible etiologies? Cardiogenic or artery-to-artery embolization is certainly possible, but the stereotypic manifestations in this patient are rather convincing for small vessel stenosis. The noncontrast CT scan ruled out hemorrhage as a cause. Workup to help determine etiology and stratify risk of subsequent stroke is paramount, which may require admission to the hospital for expedited testing. Stroke risk following a TIA can be stratified using the ABCD2 score, which can help triage who would benefit from admission (score of ≥4) or who could receive urgent completion of outpatient studies within 24–72 hours (Table 20.1).

Helpful labs include a comprehensive metabolic profile, coagulation studies, hemoglobin A1c, and lipid panel. Testing for a hypercoagulable state can also be considered if there is clinical concern, though some studies

TABLE 20.1 **ABCD2 score**

Category	+0 Points	+1 Point	+2 Points
Age ≥60 years	No	Yes	–
Initial SBP ≥140 or DBP ≥90	No	Yes	–
Clinical features of TIA	Other symptoms	Speech disturbance (no weakness)	Unilateral weakness
Symptom duration (minutes)	<10	10–59	≥60
Diabetes history	No	Yes	–

may be falsely elevated in the acute setting. A urinalysis or chest x-ray can be obtained if there is concern for recrudescence in the setting of infection (e.g., urinary tract infection or pneumonia, respectively), and a urine toxicology screen can help reveal additional stroke risk factors (e.g., stimulant use). An ECG should be performed to assess for atrial fibrillation. While in the hospital, the patient should be placed on telemetry and receive a 30-day cardiac monitor on discharge to screen for atrial fibrillation. The patient should also undergo a transthoracic echocardiogram (TTE) to evaluate for intracardiac thrombus, valvular disease, and the efficiency of the heart in case reduced cardiac outflow might contribute to this patient's symptoms. Obtaining a saline contrast "bubble" study with the TTE remains a topic of debate and should be reserved for those who may be candidates for closure of a patent foramen ovale if found.

This patient already underwent a noncontrast CT scan of his head, which can help assess for blood but does not provide information on the vessels of the head or neck. A CT angiogram of the head and neck extending to the aortic arch can show vessel stenosis or dissection. MR angiography (MRA) with gadolinium is an alternative; if the patient cannot receive gadolinium, an MRA can be performed without gadolinium using a "time of flight" sequence. Alternatively, neck vessel patency can be assessed with bilateral carotid ultrasound, but this excludes the intracranial vasculature.

Primary stroke prevention is the next consideration. A daily aspirin should be started. There are a few scenarios where dual antiplatelet therapy

(DAPT) should be considered. Patients with TIA or minor stroke—without upcoming surgery or reason for anticoagulation—are recommended to start DAPT. One approach is to start aspirin (81 mg/d) plus clopidogrel (600 mg loading dose, followed by 75 mg/d) for 21 days, with antiplatelet monotherapy thereafter. It is also recommended to start a high-dose statin with goal LDL of less than 70 mmol/L. Anticoagulation should be discussed if the patient is found to have atrial fibrillation on cardiac monitoring. Normotension should be targeted—though an exception is stated later—and blood glucose should stay within a normal range.

If the patient is determined to have symptomatic carotid stenosis (stenosis >70%), urgent treatment is recommended within the same hospitalization given the high risk of recurrent stroke. The CREST study looked at treatment of carotid stenosis by stenting (CAS) or carotid endarterectomy (CEA). Here, individual outcomes revealed a twofold higher risk of perioperative stroke with CAS compared with CEA, whereas CEA yielded a twofold higher risk of perioperative myocardial infarction. Several factors must be considered when deciding on the appropriate treatment, including the patient's medical comorbidities, age, gender, and life expectancy, as well as the degree and location of the stenosis.

If a focally stenotic MCA or MCA branch consistent with this patient's symptomatology is identified, treatment must focus on management of hypertension and any other possible risk factors including statin treatment of hyperlipidemia. However, maintenance of adequate BP may be the most helpful intervention aimed at preventing permanent ischemic damage to the territory supplied by the focally stenotic artery in the short term. This quandary is usually approached carefully by allowing BP to remain elevated to 220 mm Hg, with gradual reduction in the setting of neurologic exam checks. For symptomatic intracranial atherosclerosis, the SAMMPRIS trial demonstrated that maximal medical therapy, including DAPT with aspirin and clopidogrel for 90 days, was superior to stenting for secondary prevention of stroke. Following the 90-day period, antiplatelet monotherapy is continued. Endovascular stenting of intracranial vessels is not recommended. More aggressive antithrombotic therapy with warfarin has not proved any better than aspirin so should not be used.

Last, this is an opportunity to review lifestyle choices, such as encouraging cardiovascular exercise and cessation of tobacco products, if applicable. Stroke teaching and precautions should also be provided before discharge.

KEY POINTS TO REMEMBER

- Recurrent transient neurological symptoms are best regarded as a warning for impending cerebral ischemic damage unless proved otherwise.
- Cerebral ischemia tends to produce "negative phenomena," whereas migraine and focal epilepsy more "positive symptomatology."
- TIAs should warrant a search for the contributing arterial causes as well as risk factors for stroke, including consideration of a 30-day cardiac monitor.
- Select patients with TIA or minor stroke are recommended to start DAPT for 21 days, followed by antiplatelet monotherapy thereafter . Patients with symptomatic intracranial atherosclerosis are recommended to use DAPT for 90 days.

Further Reading

Castel J, Mlynash M, Lee K, et al. Agreement regarding diagnosis of transient ischemic attack fairly low among stroke-trained neurologists. *Stroke.* 2010;41:1367–1370.

Chimowitz MI, Lynn MJ, Derdeyn CP, et al. Stenting versus aggressive medical therapy for intracranial arterial stenosis. *N Engl J Med.* Sep 15 2011;365(11):993–1003.

Gladstone DJ, Spring M, Dorian P, et al. Atrial fibrillation in patients with cryptogenic stroke. *N Engl J Med.* Jun 26 2014;370(26):2467–2477.

Johnston SC, Rothwell PM, Nguyen-Huynh MN, et al. Validation and refinement of scores to predict very early stroke risk after transient ischaemic attack. *Lancet.* Jan 27 2007;369(9558):283–292.

Kernan WN, Ovbiagele B, Black HR, et al. Guidelines for the prevention of stroke in patients with stroke and transient ischemic attack: a guideline for healthcare professionals from the American Heart Association/American Stroke Association. *Stroke.* 2014;45(7):2160–2236.

21 Acute Neuralgia

A 65-year-old man is seen in the ED for excruciating right facial pain which has been bothering him for the past several weeks, but which escalated dramatically this morning. The most painful territory is in the right preauricular and lower cheek areas, and he is moaning and in tears due to its severity and incessancy. Pain feels "electrical" and "burning." He denies headache or pain anywhere else, and has had no changes in vision, muscle strength or coordination. He denies recent rashes or other recent illnesses. CT scan of the head is normal as is routine blood testing. Neurological exam is remarkable only for some hearing loss bilaterally and reduction in reflexes diffusely. He is resistant to any touching of the face because it exacerbates the pain, but there is no tenderness over the mastoid or areas outside the painful region. There are no skin changes noted.

What do you do now?

This patient probably has a typical case of trigeminal neuralgia (TN), which has become intractable. Pain can mount to such an extent that some patients become suicidal. Fortunately, there are some useful strategies acutely, but first, steps should be taken to rule out other causes of his pain.

TN is considered a "primary neuralgia," implying that it is not due to some underlying pathological process. This is, of course, not true, as it is probably the result of some insult to the trigeminal nerve or nucleus that has not been fully characterized. Many believe most cases of TN to be the result of compression of the proximal trigeminal nerve by an artery, often the superior cerebellar artery. At any rate, it is your responsibility to exclude other causes. Meningeal inflammatory/infectious processes, tumors, aneurysms, and abscesses can cause irritation of the trigeminal nerve, and a multiple sclerosis (MS) plaque near the root entry zone in the pons can also produce secondary trigeminal neuralgic syndromes. Herpetic infection of the nerve as well as post-herpetic neuralgia can be the cause. Inflammatory, infectious, thrombotic, granulomatous, neoplastic, and vascular lesions in the cavernous sinus can also cause a TN picture. In these cases, only the first two divisions of the trigeminal are involved at most, since the third division, the mandibular branch, does not pass through the cavernous sinus. Cluster headache, paroxysmal hemicrania (PH), and the syndrome of short-lasting unilateral neuralgiform headache (SUN) can all lead to pain that can be mistaken for TN. Cluster headaches are generally much longer than the lancinations of TN, PH and SUN headaches. PH and SUN headaches are shorter, but all three of these primary headache disorders are associated with autonomic features like tearing, rhinorrhea, and nasal congestion ipsilateral to the pain, which are not present with the presenting case. Infection or neoplastic disease in the sinus, orbit, ear or mouth can also mimic TN (Box 21.1).

A good workup for suspected TN would include brain MRI with and without contrast to exclude MS, brainstem region masses or infection, and cavernous sinus region lesions. MR angiography can be helpful to identify vascular compression of the nerve. Lumbar puncture might be indicated, particularly if there are other cranial nerves involved, to rule out an infectious, inflammatory, or neoplastic process. A search for herpetic lesions or

BOX 21.1   **Differential diagnosis of trigeminal neuralgia**

Cavernous sinus syndromes
Cluster headache
Paroxysmal hemicranias
Short-lasting unilateral neuralgiform headaches
Hemifacial spasm
Migraine headache
Post-herpetic neuralgia
Subarachnoid hemorrhage
Sinus, ocular, or otic pathology
Herpetic and post-herpetic neuralgia
Multiple sclerosis
Chronic meningeal infection/inflammation (Lyme, TB, sarcoidosis)

scars might be revealing. And a very good head and neck exam should be done to exclude an otic, orbital, or sinus lesion or infection.

Most patients with TN can get good, long-lasting relief with judicious use of antineuralgia medication such as carbamazepine, oxcarbazepine, gabapentin, amitriptyline, or baclofen, as well as a number of second-line prophylactic medications, including lamotrigine, pregabalin, and phenytoin. The use of botulinum toxin type A injected in the region of the greatest pain has been used effectively in some cases as well. Trigeminal nerve decompression is often recommended when imaging reveals vascular compression of the nerve. For intractable cases, ablative procedures of the trigeminal nerve or Gasserian ganglion (including gamma knife procedures) have been successful in some cases, though potential adverse effects, such as worsening pain due to denervation, must be considered.

However, the problem confronting you is how to stop this man's excruciating pain as soon as possible. Intravenous phenytoin has been helpful for a number of patients at a dose of 15 mg/kg infused slowly, with care taken to avoid extravascular injection as this can be highly toxic to dermal tissues (leading in some cases to the "purple glove syndrome"). Fosphenytoin is safer and, while costlier, is equally effective. Intravenous lidocaine can also be useful in a dose up to 5 mg per kilogram of body weight in 250 mL of

5% dextrose solution over 1 hour. Standard cardiac monitoring is advisable as lidocaine can induce arrhythmia. Occipital nerve blocks with lidocaine or bupivacaine have helped some patients acutely. Other parenteral anticonvulsants have been tried in the acute setting, including levetiracetam. Neuroleptic antiemetics have also been helpful for selected patients in excruciating pain from TN. Chlorpromazine, for example, at a dose of 25–50 mg IV given carefully with diphenhydramine to prevent dystonic reaction, seems to be effective in acute exacerbations of TN. This can be very sedating, so patients must be watched carefully after administration. Finally, there are reports of benefit from a number of other interventions including ocular topical anesthetic (when pain seems greatest in the ophthalmic division), sumatriptan given subcutaneously, and intravenous infusion of magnesium sulfate in the 1–3 g range. Here, too, cardiac monitoring may be wise.

TN typically produces lancinating pain and can be triggered by touch, as in this patient. The usual areas of pain fall into the maxillary and mandibular regions of the face (served by the lower two divisions of the trigeminal nerve). Patients may be seen to have contractions of their face on the side of pain (hence the synonym for TN: *tic doloroux*). This is not to be confused with hemifacial spasm, thought to be due to irritation of the facial nerve. But some patients complain of more aching type pain without the other features of TN. This has been termed "atypical facial pain" and carried the connotation of psychogenic etiology. It seems much more likely that it is simply a different manifestation of the same process—trigeminal irritation—and the search for secondary causes and successful treatment is very similar.

For those interested in the classification of neuropathic pain subtypes, the International Classification of Headache Disorders approach may help, in which consistent categories are used for neuropathic pain involving the face or head. According to this approach, *neuralgia* is used to describe primarily lancinating pain derived from a pathological process affecting the nerve, and *painful neuropathy* is used to describe pain that is generally continuous with evidence of a sensory deficit on exam (Box 21.2). This classification is generalizable to other neuralgias. Likewise, the acute and prophylactic treatment described earlier tends to be effective for other neuropathic pain conditions such as glossopharyngeal neuralgia and occipital neuralgia.

International Classification of Headache Disorders (3rd ed.)

Classification of trigeminal nerve pain

13.1 Pain attributed to a lesion or disease of the trigeminal nerve

    13.1.1 Trigeminal neuralgia

        13.1.1.1 Classical trigeminal neuralgia (due to vascular compression)

        13.1.1.2 Secondary trigeminal neuralgia (MS, masses, etc.)

        13.1.1.3 Idiopathic trigeminal neuralgia

    13.1.2 Painful trigeminal neuropathy

        13.1.2.1 Painful trigeminal neuropathy attributed to herpes zoster

        13.1.2.2 Trigeminal post-herpetic neuralgia

        13.1.2.3 Painful post-traumatic trigeminal neuropathy

        13.1.2.4 Painful trigeminal neuropathy attributed to other disorder

        13.1.2.5 Idiopathic painful trigeminal neuropathy

KEY POINTS TO REMEMBER

- Acute exacerbations of TN can be excruciating and even lead to suicidality.
- Prophylactic pharmacological treatment of TN is generally very effective.
- There are several options for acute treatment of exacerbations, with guidelines now available for guidance.
- Atypical facial pain is a somewhat perjorative term that probably represents an overlap syndrome with many features of TN.

Further Reading

Bendtsen L, Zakrzewska JM, Abbott J, et al. European Academy of Neurology guideline on trigeminal neuralgia. *Eur J Neurol.* 2019;26(6):831–849.

Cruccu G, Gronseth G, Alksne J, et al. AAN-EFNS guidelines on trigeminal neuralgia management. *Eur J Neurol.* 2008;15:1013–1028.

Headache Classification Committee of the International Headache Society (IHS). The International Classification of Headache Disorders (3rd ed.). *Cephalalgia.* 2018;38:1–211.

Moore D, Chong MS, Shetty A, Zakrzewska, JM. A systematic review of rescue
   analgesic strategies in acute exacerbations of primary trigeminal neuralgia. *Br J
   Anaesth*. 2019;123(2):e385–e396.
Newman JW, Blunck JR, Fields RK, Croom JE. Fosphenytoin-induced purple glove
   syndrome: a case report. *Clin Neurol Neurosurg*. 2017;160:50–53.

22 Intractable Migraine

A 32-year-old woman with a several year history of migraine is being seen in the ED for a severe headache which has failed to respond to IM ketorolac 60 mg, prochlorperazine 25 mg IM and lorazepam 4 mg IM. She tried sumatriptan PO at home last night, which was ineffective. She states that the pain is unbearable and beseeches you to "just give me a shot of morphine!" You see that her last ED visit for headache occurred 2 weeks ago and that she has had 9 visits to the ED in the last 6 months. She also complains of some nausea, severe photo- and phono-phobia, and some mild vertigo. She is taking amitriptyline 100 mg qhs, topiramate 100 mg bid, propranolol 80 mg bid, and clonazepam 2 mg qhs. She also takes sumatriptan, hydrocodone and butalbital as well as an assortment of over-the-counter analgesics regularly. She has a normal general exam, a supple neck, and no neurological findings. Funduscopic exam is also normal. CT of the head is normal.

What do you do now?

There is no emergency room physician who cannot recall many patients whose presentation was nearly identical to this patient's. The headache is most likely migraine, fitting the diagnosis of "status migrainosus" (Box 22.1), but making sure to rule out secondary causes of headaches is imperative. Intracranial by mass, hemorrhage, meningitis, encephalitis, hydrocephalus, and abscess are all highly unlikely with a normal exam. But cervical arterial dissection, vasculitis, reversible cerebral vasoconstriction syndrome, toxicity or metabolic derangement, cerebral venous thrombosis, and an array of less common causes of headache must be considered. A way to quickly decide whether to embark on a workup for these is to ask the following questions:

- Was the headache onset sudden (thunderclap)?
- Is this a new headache or a change from the old headache pattern?
- Is there fever, significant hypertension, or neck stiffness?
- Is there any finding on neurological exam including cognitive dysfunction?
- Is this headache occurring in the setting of systemic illness (e.g., AIDS, cancer)?

BOX 22.1   **International Classification of Headache Disorders criteria for status migrainosus**

1.4.1 Status migrainosus
Description: A debilitating migraine attack lasting for more than
    72 hours
Diagnostic criteria:
A. A headache attack fulfilling criteria B and C
B. Occurring in a patient with 1.1 Migraine without aura and/or 1.2 Migraine with aura, and typical of previous attacks except for its duration and severity
C. Both of the following characteristics:
    1. unremitting for >72 hours
    2. pain and/or associated symptoms are debilitating
D. Not better accounted for by another ICHD-3 diagnosis

Generally, the answer to all of these is No. But if any of these "red flags" are present, imaging of the head, lumbar puncture, cerebrovascular imaging, and extensive metabolic screening may be indicated.

If this is indeed simply another migraine, why is it so unresponsive to medication, and why is she having to come to the ED so often despite prophylactic medication and appropriate acute headache medication? Unfortunately, the medications are most likely contributing to this patient's problems. When migraine patients overuse analgesic and/or migraine-abortive medications, headache frequency may increase via an as yet poorly understood mechanism. Previously termed "analgesic rebound," this condition is referred to as *medication overuse headache* (MOH), and it is very challenging to treat. It is also difficult to diagnose with certainty since there are certainly patients who developed frequent migraine attacks prior to using acute medications frequently—thus the medication use is a result not a cause of the frequent headaches.

In patients with MOH, there is poor response to acute treatments, even those that were once useful. And when they try to discontinue their acute "rescue meds," pain worsens and they tend to give up. These patients also tend to lose responsiveness to prophylactic medications. The frequency and doses of the analgesic/abortive medications needed to produce this syndrome probably varies from patient to patient and with different acute medications, but usage on 3 days per week or more is generally thought to be enough to cause MOH (Box 22.2).

So, an apparently unsolvable problem confronts the medical team here. Fortunately, there are some reasonably good options for immediate control of pain that will not escalate the problem of medication overuse. Ketorolac was a good choice but was not effective, possibly because of the frequent use of OTC medications in the NSAID category. Another option is intravenous valproate which is given as a 500–1,000 mg bolus. Intravenous magnesium sulfate is another option and is given in doses of 1 g up to 5 g total as slow IV push. Intravenous dihydroergotamine (DHE) 1 mg is another option although should not be given in close temporal proximity to a triptan, as vasoconstrictive effects can be additive. Greater occipital nerve blocks seem to be very helpful for some patients, although the mechanism is not well understood.

Intravenous neuroleptic medication can be extremely useful for acute refractory migraine. A good choice is prochlorperazine 10 mg. Because of the

8.2 Medication-overuse headache (MOH): Headache on 15 or more days per month in the setting of chronic overuse of acute medications (generally >10 per month usage, but >15 days/ month for NSAIDs)

8.2.1 Ergotamine-overuse headache

8.2.2 Triptan-overuse headache

8.2.3 Non-opioid analgesic-overuse headache

    8.2.3.1 Paracetamol (acetaminophen)-overuse headache

    8.2.3.2 Non-steroidal anti-inflammatory drug (NSAID)-overuse headache

8.2.4 Opioid-overuse headache

8.2.5 Combination-analgesic-overuse headache

8.2.6 Medication-overuse headache attributed to multiple drug classes not individually overused

8.2.7 Medication-overuse headache attributed to unspecified or unverified overuse of multiple drug classes

From *International Classification of Headache Disorders* (3rd ed.).

risk of dystonia, this is often administered with diphenhydramine 25 mg intravenously. Finally, parenteral corticosteroids, either as a one-time dose or followed by a tapering oral dose over several days can break a cycle of migraine, though there tends to be some delay after initial dosing. This might consist of 1,000 mg of methylprednisolone or 6–8 mg of dexamethasone. The evidence for acute relief of migraine with steroids is weak but it does seem that they can effectively prevent recurrence of the headache when used in addition to other interventions.

Opioids are to be avoided. While they can certainly relieve pain, the effect is temporary, and large doses are generally required, leading to significant sedation. Plus, opioids will just amplify the medication overuse condition. Patients who have had opioid treatment in the past may remember the gratifying relief of pain (and perhaps euphoria) and ask for it again. This is interpreted as illicit drug-seeking, but rather, it may be better framed as appropriate protective behavior. Nonetheless, the request for opioids is to be countered with clear explanations regarding why they are not indicated. If all approaches fail, the patient can be admitted and treated more aggressively, perhaps with a course of intravenous DHE infusions or parenteral neuroleptics.

Some or all of the above are usually successful in alleviating the patient's headache or at least significantly reducing its severity. But the problem of headache recurrence, very likely in the setting of medication overuse, remains. Patients like this must be enlisted in the fight to limit acute pain medications, and it may be reasonable to refer them to a headache specialist who can simplify and adjust the prophylactic program and help to design a multimodal treatment plan.

KEY POINTS TO REMEMBER

- Even patients with a known headache disorder must be thoughtfully evaluated for the presence of a new secondary cause when presenting to the ED with intractable pain.
- There are a number of parenteral pharmacological choices for acute migraine treatment including ketorolac, DHE, magnesium, valproate, neuroleptics, and corticosteroids.
- Occipital nerve blocks may be a useful addition to the treatment options.
- Medication overuse may complicate the picture of acute refractory migraine and must be addressed.

Further Reading

Friedman BW. Review: phenothiazines relieve acute migraine headaches in the ED and are better than other active agents for some outcomes. *Ann Intern Med.* 2010;152:JC4–JC11.

Katsarava Z, Holle D, Diener H-C. Medication overuse headache. *Curr Neurol Neurosci Rep.* 2009; 9:115–119.

Marmura MJ, Silberstein SD, Schwedt TJ. The acute treatment of migraine in adults: the American Headache Society Evidence assessment of migraine pharmacotherapies. *Headache.* 2015;55(1):3–20.

Singh A, Alter HJ, Zaia B. Does the addition of dexamethasone to standard therapy for acute migraine headache decrease the incidence of recurrent headache for patients treated in the emergency department? A meta-analysis and systematic review of the literature. *Acad Emerg Med.* 2008;15(12):1223–1233.

23 Intracerebral Hemorrhage on Anticoagulation

A 66-year-old man with a history of atrial fibrillation and myocardial infarction complicated by heart failure was admitted to the hospital for ventricular assist device placement, now on a therapeutic heparin infusion. His hospital course was also complicated by acute on chronic renal failure, requiring continuous renal replacement therapy. While working with physical therapy he is noted to be newly confused and not moving his right side. A stroke alert is called. His vital signs include a blood pressure (BP) of 90/50, pulse 95. His finger-stick blood glucose is 110. His pupils are symmetric and reactive. His NIH Stroke Scale is 24, notable for global aphasia, left gaze preference, right field cut, right facial weakness, right hemiparesis, and sensory loss. He is emergently intubated for airway protection and taken for a noncontrast head CT, which shows a large left frontal intracerebral hemorrhage (ICH) with midline shift.

What do you do now?

Even before the head CT is obtained, there is high concern for an ICH given his rapid clinical deterioration, his focal neurologic deficits on exam, and the important history of concurrent anticoagulation use. ICH carries a high rate of disability and mortality, and patients with ICH are at risk of early decompensation from hematoma expansion, so it is important to act quickly. In these situations, there are several things to keep in mind before the patient leaves the unit for head imaging. The first thing is to ensure that the patient is stable enough to go to the CT scanner, which includes lying flat for several minutes. If intubation is indicated, try to obtain a rapid neurologic exam prior to the use of paralytics in order to guide initial management.

Depending on the patient's history, exam, and clinical circumstance, it may be reasonable to begin treatment for increased intracranial pressure prior to obtaining the head CT, as discussed later. In addition to a noncontrast head CT (see Figures 23.1 and 23.2), which will quickly provide information on the presence of blood or cerebral edema, it is often helpful to also obtain a CT angiogram (CTA) of the brain. The CTA will help determine whether the ICH is from a vascular cause, like an aneurysm or vascular malformation. For example, hemorrhage involving the sylvian fissure is often aneurysmal in origin. Contrast enhancement within the ICH ("spot sign") may indicate active bleeding. CT venogram (CTV) should also be considered as a significant minority of venous occlusions present with hemorrhage.

ICH is often complicated by increased intracranial pressure (ICP), which requires emergent identification and treatment. Management of increased ICP centers on the Monroe-Kelli doctrine, which states that any sudden change in volume of the different intracranial compartments—broadly speaking, parenchyma, blood, and CSF—will result in increased ICP due to the fixed volume of the skull. Immediate steps can be taken at the bedside, including elevating the head of the bed and ensuring the head is midline, to encourage venous return. Temporary hyperventilation ($PaCO_2$ goal of 30–35 mm Hg) with gradual reversal, either through bag-masking or intubation, leads to arterial vasoconstriction and so lowers cerebral blood volume and ICP. If possible, a reduction in positive end-expiratory pressure (PEEP) can reduce intrathoracic pressure, facilitating venous return. Hyperosmolar therapy, either with mannitol or hypertonic (23.4%) saline,

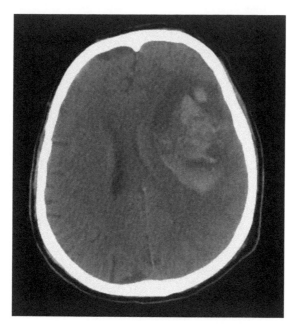

FIGURE 23.1 Noncontrast CT of the head showing large left frontal parenchymal hematoma with mass effect.

can be given. At this time, there is no clear evidence of superiority of one agent over the other and so the choice is often determined by accessibility and expediency. Serum sodium and osmolality should be trended with a goal of hypernatremia (serum sodium approximately 145–155 mEq/L) and hyperosmolality (300–320 mosmol/kg). Hypotonic fluids should be avoided.

Any coagulopathy in someone with ICH should be emergently reversed, if the benefits outweigh the risks. Coagulopathy may be iatrogenic, hereditary, or acquired from a systemic process (e.g., malignancy, uremia). For patients on an unfractionated heparin infusion, IV protamine sulfate can be given for reversal, with a dose based on the amount of heparin received and the timing of its last administration. For patients on warfarin, the INR will serve as a guide for reversal with a goal of INR lower than 1.5. If the anticoagulation is iatrogenic, is important to keep in mind the reason for starting it in the first place and what the risks of reversal may be, but expedited reversal remains paramount.

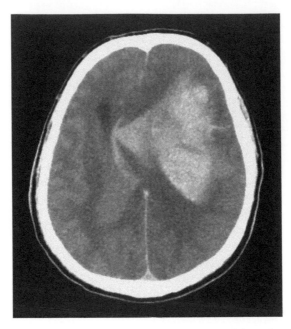

FIGURE 23.2 CT of the same left frontal parenchymal hematoma with interval expansion 6 hours later.

In order to reverse vitamin K antagonist (e.g., warfarin), an INR will serve as the guide for four-factor prothrombin complex concentrate (PCC) administration, which is favored over fresh frozen plasma. Vitamin K 10 mg IV should also be provided over 30 minutes with close monitoring, given risk for anaphylaxis. Direct oral anticoagulants have several benefits over warfarin as anticoagulants but are more challenging to reverse. If the last dose was given within 2 hours, activated charcoal can be given to reduce absorption. The reversal agent for dabigatran is idarucizumab. The reversal agent for apixaban and rivaroxaban is andexanet alfa.

If a patient is receiving tissue plasminogen activator (tPA) and experiences an acute neurologic decline, a stat noncontrast head CT should be obtained to assess for hemorrhage. In patients with suspected hemorrhage, the tPA infusion should be stopped. Treatment options in this scenario include cryoprecipitate 10 units or the use of antifibrinolytic agents, such as aminocaproic acid or tranexamic acid.

Platelet transfusions may be helpful if the patient is thrombocytopenic (platelet <100,000/µL). However, platelet transfusions are not indicated—and may even be harmful—if the goal is to "reverse" recent antiplatelet use, as shown in the PATCH trial.

Neurosurgical colleagues should also be consulted immediately. Rapid correction of a coagulopathy will also prevent delay of surgical intervention if needed. An external ventricular drain (EVD; also known as ventriculostomy or extraventricular drain) should be considered if there is hydrocephalus or significant intraventricular hemorrhage from a supratentorial hemorrhage. Decompressive hemicraniectomy should be discussed for large ICH, especially cerebellar hemorrhages larger than 3 cm, as these increase the risk of brainstem compression and ventricular obstruction leading to acute hydrocephalus.

The management of refractory elevated ICP centers on the reduction of brain metabolism and improved ventilator synchrony with the use of sedation and paralytics.

Unlike this scenario, intraparenchymal hemorrhage is often accompanied by hypertension because of uncontrolled chronic hypertension as a cause for the hemorrhage or as a stress response. In severe cases, hypertension is accompanied by bradycardia and irregular breathing, which is the Cushing response seen with increased intracranial pressure. Common areas of hemorrhage seen with hypertensive bleeds are the basal ganglia, thalamus, pons, and cerebellum. When faced with a hypertensive patient, current evidence suggests that a rapid reduction in BP can reduce the risk of hematoma expansion and improve outcomes. The BP target is an area of controversy. Recent guidelines recommend that if the systolic BP (SBP) is between 150 and 220 mm Hg and there is no contraindication to acute BP treatment, then acute lowering to SBP 140 mm Hg is safe and can improve functional outcome. The choice of antihypertensive is also important as venodilators may increase ICP. Overaggressive BP reduction, below the recommended target, can result in ischemia and increased edema, especially in patients with a long-standing history of hypertension.

Clinical seizures should be treated with antiepileptics. However, in nontraumatic ICH, there are no data to support the use of prophylactic antiepileptics. Similarly, there is no evidence to support steroid use for cerebral edema in these cases.

Even before the patient is stabilized, prognostication of neurologic outcome will likely come up. The latest American Heart Association/American Stroke Association (AHA/ASA) guidelines caution providing early prognostication because current models are insufficient. For this reason, these guidelines encourage early aggressive care and postponement of a new do-not-resuscitate (DNR) order until at least the second full hospitalization day.

KEY POINTS TO REMEMBER

- In addition to a noncontrast head CT, consider the use of vessel imaging (arterial and venous) to assess for alternate etiologies of hemorrhage.
- Treatment of coagulopathy is specific to the underlying cause. Platelets are not indicated unless the patient is thrombocytopenic (platelet <100,000/μL).
- Be on the lookout for signs of increased ICP and treat expeditiously.
- An external ventricular drain may be needed if there is significant intraventricular blood or hydrocephalus.

Further Reading

Baharoglu MI, Cordonnier C, Al-Shahi Salman R, et al. Platelet transfusion versus standard care after acute stroke due to spontaneous cerebral haemorrhage associated with antiplatelet therapy (PATCH): a randomised, open-label, phase 3 trial. *Lancet.* 2016;387(10038):2605–2613.

Hemphill JC, 3rd, Greenberg SM, Anderson CS, et al. Guidelines for the Management of Spontaneous Intracerebral Hemorrhage: A Guideline for Healthcare Professionals From the American Heart Association/American Stroke Association. *Stroke.* 2015;46(7):2032–2060.

Witt DM, Nieuwlaat R, Clark NP, et al. American Society of Hematology 2018 guidelines for management of venous thromboembolism: optimal management of anticoagulation therapy. *Blood Adv.* 2018;2(22):3257–3291.

24 First Seizure

A 42-year-old man was seen earlier today to "look off into space" and, within a few minutes, was observed to have a generalized rhythmic shaking of his legs and arms. He had urinary incontinence. He has had no recent illnesses or medical symptoms. He has been working a second job lately—and sleeping less—due to financial need. He has no history of seizures or stroke. CT of the head was normal as was a lumbar puncture. He is very anxious. Vital signs are normal except for tachycardia at 110. Blood count reveals a WBC of 12,000, but RBC count, hematocrit, and hemoglobin are normal as are serum chemistries. Full neurological exam is entirely normal.

What do you do now?

The first question in a patient with a first-time seizure-like spell is: "Is this epileptic?" It certainly sounds like it here, but it is important to remember that there a number of conditions which can mimic seizures including movement disorders, TIA, syncope, psychiatric conditions, and migraine. None of these seems likely here.

When patients do not recover from their seizure completely, have a prolonged postictal period (more than a couple of hours), have multiple seizures, are sick medically, or have an unstable/unsupervised home life, hospitalization is warranted. This patient, who apparently has none of these complicating issues, will probably be anxious to return home, which is not unreasonable. But the neurologist, who may never see this patient again, has a responsibility to attempt to predict the future here and do everything possible to rule out treatable causes of seizures and prevent their recurrence.

The WBC elevation is entirely expected, as generalized seizures lead to WBC demargination and spuriously increased WBC counts, but infections should be considered. Other etiological factors should be entertained such as intracranial mass lesions, meningitis, encephalitis, electrolyte imbalance (such as hyponatremia, hyper- or hypoglycmeia, hypomagnesemia, or hypocalcemia), medication side effects (opioids, antidepressants), intoxication (particularly with stimulants), or withdrawal (see Box 24.1). Here, again, none of these seems likely. Sleep deprivation is likely to have contributed. Autoimmune diseases of the brain, genetic diseases, perinatal cortical injury, and the remote effects of brain trauma are possibilities. To be certain no causative factors have been missed, the patient should have an MRI of the brain with and without contrast and an EEG with provocative maneuvers like photic stimulation and hyperventilation. Both of these can generally be done safely during the subsequent several days on an outpatient basis. After normal CT imaging of the brain, lumbar puncture is warranted in patients with fever, meningismus, or focality on neurological exam, including persistent alteration in mental status.

The decision about starting anticonvulsant medication in a patient who had a first seizure revolves around the risk of seizure recurrence, which is probably around 30% in the next 5 years, but changes depending on risk factors. One risk factor for seizure recurrence is partial onset—and here there seems to have been complex partial seizure activity (impaired awareness) followed by secondary generalization. Other risk factors are the

BOX 24.1 **Causes of first-time seizures**

Intracranial neoplasm
Subdural hematoma
Cerebral infarction
Intracerebral hemorrhage
Cerebral venous thrombosis
Cerebral vasculitis
Meningitis
Encephalitis
Brain abscess
Electrolyte imbalance (such as hyponatremia, hypomagnesemia,
    hypocalcemia, hypoglycemia or hyperglycemia, uremia)
Medication side effects (opioids, antidepressants)
Drug intoxication (amphetamines, cocaine)
Drug withdrawal (barbiturates, benzodiazepines)
Ethanol withdrawal
Perinatal cortical injury
Posttraumatic cortical injury
Inherited metabolic diseases

presence of focal neurological deficits on exam, the presence of epileptiform activity on EEG, and brain CT or MRI abnormalities. With normal MRI, the risk of a recurrence after the first seizure goes down to about 30%. Unprovoked seizures are more likely than provoked seizures to recur, but the nature of provocation is probably important. Unprovoked seizures will have highest recurrence in the first 2 years, and early antiseizure treatment is felt to be important.

Other considerations are, of course, the relative risks and benefits of anticonvulsant medication for the particular patient. The risk of antiseizure drug adverse effects is high—up to around 30%, though most of these are mild and reversible. Some neurologists ask patients about their lifestyle risks (i.e., the *consequences* of a seizure recurrence). For example, a seizure recurrence in a long-distance truck driver might be of more concern than in an office worker. However, *any* generalized seizure is potentially life-threatening, particularly if it should happen while the patient is driving, on a stairway, etc. Therefore, the decision is individual and should be made as a team with input from the patient, family, and neurologist. Often, if workup is entirely normal, instituting anticonvulsant therapy is done with the plan of tapering and stopping medication within a year if seizures have not recurred and EEG remains normal. This might be reasonable here. Equally reasonable, if the patient wishes, the decision can be postponed until the EEG and further brain imaging has been done. And it is not unreasonable to simply choose to adjust lifestyle to raise the seizure "threshold" and avoid taking anticonvulsants entirely for the time being. For this patient this would involve assuring adequate sleep, avoiding intoxicants like ethanol, and probably looking into stress-reducing tactics including personal counseling. Most neurologists would agree that anticonvulsant treatment is indicated after two seizures as recurrence risk is significantly higher after two or more unprovoked seizures than after just one, rising to 70% even in patients with normal brain MRI scans.

The best choice in anticonvulsant medication for a first-time generalized seizure is not clear. Several studies have attempted to compare the available anticonvulsants on the basis of effectiveness and tolerance, but different results seem to surface. All antiepileptic drugs can potentially have fairly significant side effects, and many alter hepatic metabolic activity. Some should be titrated upward slowly, which will lead to a delay in attaining therapeutic levels. Serum drug concentrations can be useful with some anticonvulsants but not all.

Since little is yet known about this patient's seizure type other than it became generalized, a good choice might be to begin with a medication that is good for seizures with an unknown classification. It is essential to know and share with patients the common adverse effects of the AEDs you are considering and what monitoring lab tests will be necessary.

It is worth letting patients know that around 10% of people will have one seizure, about 1% have epilepsy (more than two unprovoked seizures), but, having had one seizure, there is a higher risk of having a second seizure.

Based on this, many patients will opt to start an AED, at least for several months. Whatever is decided, the patient should be cautioned about risks of driving, operating machinery, or doing any activity that might be dangerous to himself or others if he were to have a seizure. You should be aware of state laws concerning cessation of driving after documented seizure occurrence and counsel the patient about his or her responsibilities concerning this as well as any requirement for you to notify state motor vehicle departments.

KEY POINTS TO REMEMBER

- First-time seizures should trigger a workup to exclude intracranial pathology and metabolic causes.
- The acute evaluation of a patient with a first-time seizure should include CT scan of the brain, and preferably, EEG, as well as full metabolic evaluation including toxicology.
- LP should be performed if there is concern for meningitis or encephalitis.
- MRI of the brain should also be completed in the near future.
- The decision to begin seizure prophylaxis depends on the patient's risks, preferences, and results of the workup, particularly MRI and EEG.

Further Reading

Bao EL, Chao LY, Ni P, et al. Antiepileptic drug treatment after an unprovoked first seizure: a decision analysis. *Neurology.* 2018;91(15):e1429–e1439.

Bonnet LJ, Shukralla A, Tudur-Smith C, Williamson PR, Marson AG. Seizure recurrence after antiepileptic drug withdrawal and the implications for driving: further results from the MRC Antiepileptic Drug Withdrawal Study and a systematic review. *J Neurol Neurosurg Psychiatry.* 2011;82:1328–1333.

Faught E. The cost of the second seizure: rethinking the treatment decision. *Epilepsy Curr.* 2019;19(2):88–90.

25 Acute Stroke Up to 24 Hours

A 61-year-old man with untreated hypertension woke up with difficulty moving his right arm and difficulty speaking. He went to bed at approximately 10 pm and awoke to these symptoms at 6 am. Both symptoms have persisted. His wife called the paramedics, who activated a stroke alert in the field. The patient is alert but is unable to follow verbal commands or speak. He has decreased movement of the lower right face and is unable to move his right arm. Paresis is noted in the right deltoid, triceps, biceps, wrist extensors, and finger extensors. The right leg is also weak but not as severely. Sensation seems intact to noxious stimulation. His coordination appears intact on the left. CT of the head is negative, ECG shows sinus rhythm without any signs of cardiac ischemia. His wife pleads with you to do something as he is a carpenter and they are very worried about a disabling stroke.

What do you do now?

As a neurology trainee, there were few scenarios more disappointing than determining that someone with an acute stroke was out of the window for treatment. This was especially true for those who "woke up" with stroke symptoms and so often fell outside the previously narrow 6-hour eligibility limit for endovascular thrombectomy. Now, therapeutic options for acute stroke have expanded in the past few years, rendering thrombectomy available to more patients than ever before.

There are several key pieces of information that are needed when an acute stroke is suspected before considering treatment. First you must establish when the patient was last known to be at his or her neurologic baseline. This gives the best estimate of when the stroke began and is distinct from when the patient may have been found down or with a new deficit. *Don't forget to ask the patient.* However, if the patient cannot participate or is aphasic, this information may need to come from family, friends, or bystanders. Two large-bore IVs should be placed (these will be needed if antihypertensives, contrast, or thrombolytics are given). Stat labs should include chemistry, CBC, and coagulation profiles. A finger-stick glucose is needed to exclude hypoglycemia (glucose <50) as a stroke mimic. As part of standard protocol, patients should be weighed, and blood pressure should be controlled to less than 185/110 if the patient may be eligible for tissue plasminogen activator (tPA, alteplase), which will be discussed in more detail later.

Keep in mind that all this is occurring while the patient is being examined using the NIH Stroke Scale (NIHSS). Once the ABCs (airway, breathing, and circulation) are deemed stable, the patient should go immediately for a noncontrast head CT, CT angiography (CTA) head/neck, and CT perfusion if available.

The main goal of the noncontrast head CT is to exclude hemorrhage (see Figure 25.1). Once hemorrhage is excluded, the decision to give or withhold tPA should be made. TPA is not FDA-approved for use in the United States in a stroke of longer than 3 hours duration. However, this window was widened to 4.5 hours following the third European Cooperative Acute Stroke Study (ECASS III) that showed a higher percentage of patients with favorable outcomes if given tPA compared with placebo without difference in mortality. At the time of this publication, tPA eligibility is based on time from symptom onset rather than imaging characteristics, though this is likely to change in future.

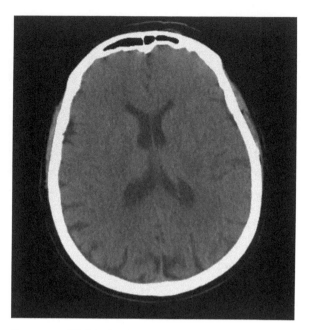

FIGURE 25.1 Noncontrast CT of the head with a loss of gray–white matter differentiation in the left insula, frontal and temporal lobes.

After the noncontrast head CT is obtained and the tPA decision is made, obtain the CTA head and neck to look for a large vessel occlusion. Unless clearly contraindicated, we *do not* wait for the creatinine to return before completing the CTA. If available, it is also important to obtain CT perfusion, which helps to differentiate brain tissue at risk (penumbra) from infarcted tissue (infarct core) (see Figures 25.2). The DAWN and DEFUSE-3 trials demonstrated efficacy of thrombectomy in patients with proximal anterior circulation occlusion up to 24 hours from symptom onset based on clinical and imaging criteria—specifically, finding patients with a large amount of tissue at risk (penumbra) but with a small infarct core.

Endovascular therapy should be pursued, regardless of whether tPA is given, for all acute ischemic strokes with distal inferior cerebral artery (ICA) or proximal middle (MCA) or anterior (ACA) occlusions. The decision to provide tPA is independent of the decision for thrombectomy, and vice versa. Symptomatic basilar thrombosis should almost always receive endovascular therapy. The efficacy of endovascular therapy was confirmed

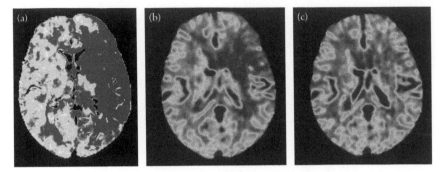

FIGURE 25.2 (a) Perfusion imaging of same lesion showing increased mean transit time. (b) Perfusion imaging of same lesion showing decreased cerebral blood flow. (c) Perfusion imaging of same lesion showing relatively preserved cerebral blood volume.

with the release of four pivotal randomized controlled trials (MR CLEAN, ESCAPE, EXTEND-IA, and SWIFT PRIME) that demonstrated improved functional outcomes at 90 days. Patients with a large-vessel occlusion should be transferred to the nearest center offering thrombectomy. In these cases, tPA can be offered prior to transfer if eligible ("drip and ship"). Optimization of the acute management of ischemic stroke is an area of neurology that is advancing rapidly and so it is important to remain vigilant for such advances.

KEY POINTS TO REMEMBER

- While IV tPA can be offered to select patients up to 4.5 hours from stroke onset, early administration is better ("time is brain").
- Thrombectomy can be offered to select patients with large-vessel occlusion up to 24 hours from symptom onset.
- Patients who are eligible for IV tPA and thrombectomy should still receive IV tPA prior to thrombectomy. If the patient must be transferred to another institution for thrombectomy, tPA can often be given prior to transfer ("drip and ship").

Further Reading

Adams, HP, del Zoppo, G, Alberts, MJ. Guidelines for the early management of adults
    with ischemic stroke. A guideline from the American Heart Association/ American
    Stroke Association Stroke Council, Clinical Cardiology Council, Cardiovascular
    Radiology and Intervention Council, and the Atherosclerotic Peripheral Vascular
    Disease and Quality of Care Outcomes in Research Interdisciplinary Working
    Groups. *Stroke.* 2007;38:1655–1711.
Albers GW, Lansberg MG, Kemp S, et al. A multicenter randomized controlled trial of
    endovascular therapy following imaging evaluation for ischemic stroke (DEFUSE
    3). *Int J Stroke.* 2017;12(8):896–905.
Hacke W, Kaste M, Bluhmki E, et al.; ECASS Investigators. Thrombolysis
    with alteplase 3 to 4.5 hours after acute ischemic stroke. *N Engl J Med.*
    2008;359:1317–1329.
Nogueira RG, Jadhav AP, Haussen DC, et al. Thrombectomy 6 to 24 hours after stroke
    with a mismatch between deficit and infarct. *N Engl J Med.* 2018;378:11–21.
Powers WJ, Rabinstein AA, Ackerson T, et al. Guidelines for the early management
    of patients with acute ischemic stroke: 2019 update to the 2018 Guidelines for
    the Early Management of Acute Ischemic Stroke: A Guideline for Healthcare
    Professionals from the American Heart Association/American Stroke Association.
    Stroke. 2019;50(12):e344–e418.

26 Acute Cervical Radiculopathy

A 52-year-old right-handed man was awakened by severe right shoulder and medial scapular pain which did not respond to ibuprofen or heat. He went to one of his twice weekly martial arts classes the night before but does not recall any specific trauma. He recalls similar pain for short periods in the last few months, but of much milder intensity. He required 2 mg of hydromorphone intravenously for relief. He endorses feeling weak in his legs transiently. He denies bladder or bowel difficulty. Left biceps and brachioradialis seem stronger than right. Right biceps reflex is diminished; otherwise reflexes are normal and there is no Babinski reflex. Abdominal reflexes are normal as are cremasteric reflexes. Gait is normal. Spurling maneuver seems to duplicate pain on the right side when looking up and to the right. Plain x-rays of the neck reveal some "mild degenerative changes" at C5-6 and C6-7, and "spine straightening". Severe pain begins to reemerge.

What do you do now?

This patient's symptoms seem to emanate from the right C6 spinal nerve, producing the characteristic shoulder and lateral arm pain. Presumably this is due to disc rupture on the basis of his recent neck stress during martial arts training. Interestingly, many patients with C6 radiculopathy seem to upper back or shoulder pain even before neck and arm pain. The cause of this is unknown but may relate to compression of the medial branches of the dorsal rami of the spinal nerves. The cervical spinal nerves originate as the dorsal and ventral roots which merge and exit at the intervertebral foramen. The spinal nerves of the neck exit the intervertebral foramen above the numbered cervical vertebrae (thoracic and lumbar nerves exit the intervertebral below the numbered vertebra). So here we will be looking for evidence of pathology in the vicinity of the C5–6 interspace. Cervical spine straightening on plain x-rays is not particularly helpful, nor is the evidence of early degenerative spine disease. MRI of the cervical spine will be important to confirm our impression of disc rupture and to rule out fracture or mass, as well as the presence of disc fragments in the spinal canal. Electromyography can be helpful at localizing the site of the pathology, but since it can be falsely normal acutely and does not provide information on the possible cause, MRI is actually superior.

Rupture of cervical intervertebral discs is less common than in lumbar discs, which is interesting because it has been shown that the annulus fibrosis in cervical discs is less robust (anatomical cadaver dissection work by Bogduk). Trauma is usually required but patients often cannot specify dramatic injuries. In our patient, as is fairly typical, subtle trauma becomes symptomatic after a bit of a delay, perhaps because the leak of nucleus pulposis material is gradual. This may underlie our patient's previous "premonitory" symptoms. Nonetheless, the pain can be intense.

Other than the pain, it is important to try to characterize the clinical state for a couple of important reasons. First, unlike lumbar disc rupture, cervical disc rupture carries the risk of spinal cord compression which, while uncommon, can lead to significant permanent myelopathy. This patient seemed to have some initial leg weakness but on exam is entirely free of myelopathic symptoms such as trunk or lower extremity sensation change, balance issues, and bowel/bladder dysfunction, and he is likewise not manifesting myelopathic findings such as hyperreflexia, increased tone, or lower extremity weakness. Intact abdominal reflexes are a nice confirmatory finding, as is the cremaster reflex. However, there can be a delay in myelopathic features, and it is wise to admit these patients for inpatient observation and surgical decompression in a timely fashion should it become necessary.

Another reason for a careful exam is to try to accurately gauge motor weakness in radicular compression. If this is minor, strength and reflexes tend to improve with conservative management, including physical therapeutic measures and pain control. But if there is significant weakness, surgical intervention may be appropriate. The surgical treatments include the anterior approach discectomy with fusion or other spine stabilizing techniques including implanted "cages." Posterior approaches, including endoscopic procedures, are gaining popularity in some areas as they do not require spine stabilization, but their outcome data are less clear. Epidural steroid infusion can help modulate pain but these seem not to provide added long-term benefit. Chiropractic manipulation has not been conclusively shown to help, and there is risk of vertebral artery injury in the high-speed manipulations practiced by many chiropractors.

KEY POINTS TO REMEMBER

- Cervical radiculopathy is often post-traumatic, but the injury can be relatively innocuous.
- C6 and C7 radicular pain can begin in the upper back and shoulder.
- Careful examination is essential to rule out myelopathy.
- MRI of the cervical spine is the best confirmatory test and is important in ruling out impending spinal cord compression, mass lesions, and spinal canal bone fragments.
- Physical therapy helps the majority of cases, but surgical disc removal may be necessary, particularly in cases of significant weakness or severe pain refractory to treatment.

Further Reading

Mehren C, Wanke-Jellinek L. Posterior foraminotomy for lateral cervical disc herniation. *Eur Spine J.* 2019;28(1):1–2.

Mizutamari M, Sei A, Tokiyoshi A, Fujimoto T, Taniwaki T, Togami W, Mizuta
H. Corresponding scapular pain with the nerve root involved in cervical
radiculopathy. *J Orthop Surg*. 2010;18(3):356–360.

Vleggeert-Lankamp CL, Janssen TM, van Zwet E, Goedmakers CM, Bosscher L,
Peul W, Arts MP. The NECK trial: effectiveness of anterior cervical discectomy
with or without interbody fusion and arthroplasty in the treatment of cervical
disc herniation; a double-blinded randomized controlled trial. *Spine J*.
2019;19(6):965–975.

27 Post-Cardiac Arrest Management

A 38-year-old man in excellent health is found unresponsive by his spouse when he fails to turn off his morning alarm. Paramedics find the patient in ventricular fibrillation; he is subsequently shocked and receives epinephrine with a conversion to pulseless electrical activity. The man is shocked again, receives additional epinephrine, with return of spontaneous circulation. He is intubated in the field with paralytics, and total CPR time is approximately 20 minutes. On arrival to the ED, blood pressure (BP) is 158/98 (without vasopressors), heart rate is 90, oxygen is 98% ventilated. Neurological exam is limited by recent use of paralytics; pupils are 3 mm and reactive bilaterally. Labs are notable for WBC 20, lactate 7, and venous blood gas with pH 7.2.

What do you do now?

After stabilization, one of the main decisions to make for this individual is whether or not to provide targeted temperature management (TTM), also known as therapeutic hypothermia or cooling. TTM is currently the only therapy shown to improve outcomes for hypoxic-ischemic neurologic injury after cardiac arrest. The randomized controlled trials that support the use of TTM only included patients with cardiac arrest in the community, although TTM may also be considered for in-hospital cardiac arrest. While previously studied in patients with cardiac arrest with shockable rhythms (ventricular fibrillation or pulseless ventricular tachycardia), there is also growing evidence to support the use of TTM following nonshockable rhythms (pulseless electrical activity or asystole) as well. For this reason, the initial cardiac rhythm does not factor into the TTM decision or subsequent prognostication.

Current guidelines recommend achieving a target temperature of 33–36°C for 24 hours, followed by 48 hours of normothermia with fever prevention. The goal is to achieve the target temperature as soon as possible. TTM is only suitable for patients who are not following commands, including patients whose exam may be clouded by sedatives and paralytics. Make your TTM decision based on what you see, not what you think the patient is capable of doing. Potential contraindications to TTM include active bleeding (especially at a noncompressible site) or an inability to maintain SBP at greater than 90 mm Hg with pressors. Acute coronary syndrome or planned cardiac interventions, including those that may require thrombolysis or anticoagulation, are *not* contraindications. If a patient is determined to be too unstable for TTM, then it is recommended to at least avoid fever for protection against neurologic deterioration.

Passive cooling can begin immediately in eligible patients with the use of surface ice packs and intravenous chilled normal saline. There are several methods for maintaining hypothermia, and so reference the protocol at your institution.

The initial neurological exam should focus on mental status, brainstem reflexes (pupil reactivity, corneal reflex, oculocephalic reflex, presence of cough and gag), and the best motor response to central and peripheral noxious stimulation.

After stabilization, a noncontrast head CT should be obtained to ensure that the cardiac arrest was not caused by an aneurysmal subarachnoid hemorrhage or other intracranial pathology. It can also be helpful to assess for presence of cerebral edema (see Figure 27.1), which can affect intracranial pressure management.

During the period of TTM maintenance, there are several aspects to monitor in addition to the core temperature. Shivering should be treated as it increases the metabolic rate and may make maintaining the goal temperature challenging. Options for shivering control include buspirone, meperidine, magnesium sulfate, benzodiazepines, and propofol. If these medications fail to adequately control shivering, paralysis can be used, but this significantly limits the exam. The patient should remain NPO and goal blood glucose is less than 180. Potassium should be replaced only up to 3.4 mEq/L as rewarming can cause rebound hyperkalemia.

Rewarming begins 24 hours from TTM start, not from when goal temperature was reached. Rewarming should occur slowly, with a temperature increase no greater than 0.5°C per hour, and then maintained at 37°C for the first 24 hours post-TTM to avoid rebound hyperthermia. Following

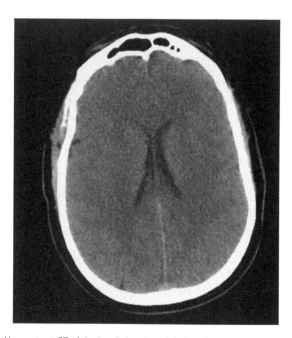

FIGURE 27.1 Noncontrast CT of the head showing global cerebral edema.

the acute period, it is recommended to maintain a core temperature of less than 37.5°C. Secondary neurologic injury can be avoided by aggressively treating fever (goal temp < 37.5°C), hypocapnia (goal $PaCO_2$ > 35 mm Hg), hyperoxemia (goal PaO_2 < 200 mm Hg), and treating seizure if present.

If, after rewarming, the patient is following commands, prognosis is excellent.

However, if the patient remains unresponsive, the question of prognostication arises. Variables used for prognostication should predict with high specificity who will have an invariably poor prognosis, to make sure that those who are labeled as having a poor prognosis have no chance of a meaningful recovery.

American Academy of Neurology (AAN) evidence-based algorithm for prognostication after cardiac arrest is based on data from the pre-TTM era. For this reason, prognostication using these guidelines must be used with caution in those who underwent TTM.

No neurologic prognostication should occur until at least 24 hours post-arrest. In those who undergo TTM, prognostication may take even longer, since hypothermia can directly affect mental status and the metabolism of drugs. Patients who undergo TTM may also receive more sedating medications than those who are not made hypothermic. It is absolutely crucial to not rush into prognostication.

The neurologic exam should be performed 72 hours post-arrest, ensuring sedatives have been discontinued for a sufficient period of time so as to not affect the examination. The examination should center on the same aspects listed earlier. In addition, quantitative pupillometry is a helpful tool when assessing pupillary reactivity.

EEG and SSEPs should be obtained after rewarming, between 24 and 72 hours post-arrest. Some institutions also recommend the use of EEG during the cooling and rewarming phases. Serum neuron specific enolase (NSE) can be measured at 48, and 72 hours post-arrest. The 72-hour exam, presence of myoclonus, NSE levels, EEG characteristics, and SSEP responses can be combined for multimodal prognostication of poor outcome. It is important to note that outcome is often described as a Cerebral Performance Category (CPC) from 1 (normal) to 5 (death). A poor outcome may group CPC 3–5, where CPC 3 refers to severe disability with dependency, but with some ability to communicate or even ambulate. For this reason, what a study labels as a poor outcome may not actually be unacceptable to a patient or surrogate decision-maker and is a significant limitation in prognostication discussions.

KEY POINTS TO REMEMBER

- Patients who do not follow commands after cardiac arrest should be considered for TTM.
- If eligible, TTM should be initiated on arrival and not delayed for procedures.
- Shivering and fever should be aggressively treated in order to reduce metabolic demands.
- No neurologic prognostication should occur until at least 24 hours post-arrest. Prognostication guidelines are largely based on pre-TTM data. In these studies, definitions of a poor/unfavorable outcome may differ from what is an acceptable quality of life to the patient's previously stated wishes or determination by decision-makers.

Further Reading

Callaway CW, Soar J, Aibiki M, et al. Part 4: Advanced life support: 2015 International consensus on cardiopulmonary resuscitation and emergency cardiovascular care science with treatment recommendations. *Circulation.* 2015;132(16 Suppl 1):S84–S145.

Geocadin RG, Callaway CW, Fink EL, et al. Standards for studies of neurological prognostication in comatose survivors of cardiac arrest: a scientific statement from the American Heart Association. *Circulation.* 2019;140(9):e517–e542.

Hawkes MA, Rabinstein AA. Neurological prognostication after cardiac arrest in the era of target temperature management. *Curr Neurol Neurosci Rep.* 2019;19(2):10.

28 Myasthenic Crisis

A 60-year-old woman with generalized myasthenia gravis presents to the ED in respiratory distress. She takes low-dose prednisone, pyridostigmine, and azathioprine. She developed congestion and cough 1 week ago. When you assess her, her heart rate is 120s, respiratory rate is 20s, oxygen saturation 88% on room air. Bedside forced vital capacity (FVC) is 0.6 L, and mean inspiratory force (MIF) is −26 cm H_2O. She is tachypneic, using accessory muscles for breathing. Her mental status is normal, but she can only speak a few words at a time. She has bilateral ptosis and bifacial weakness. Her speech is hoarse. She can barely lift her head off the pillow, and she has deltoid weakness; otherwise strength is full. The remainder of the neurologic exam is unremarkable. Labs show normal chemistries and a mild leukocytosis. Serial venous blood gases show her carbon dioxide is uptrending. A chest x-ray shows a right lower lobe opacity concerning for pneumonia.

What do you do now?

While there are many causes of respiratory distress, neuromuscular weakness is an important addition to the differential. The pneumonia is clearly not helping this patient, but her breathing difficulties are due to much more than a lung infection.

There are several bedside surrogates for respiratory strength, especially in patients with neuromuscular weakness, such as from myasthenia gravis. For example, this patient has difficulty speaking in complete sentences and she has neck flexion weakness. Neck flexion weakness is a good surrogate for diaphragmatic weakness. Neck flexion requires the accessory nerve as well as the cervical nerves arising from C2 and C3. Similarly, the diaphragm relies on the phrenic nerve, which arises from a combination of C3, C4, and C5 nerve fibers—you may recall the rhyme "C3, 4, 5 keeps the diaphragm alive." Neck flexion strength is an easy exam maneuver that can be serially monitored with each intervention. Patients may also exhibit accessory muscle use or paradoxical abdominal breathing when in respiratory distress. However, increased fatigue can make it difficult for the patient to adapt in this way, and so its absence can be falsely reassuring to the medical team.

Not all respiratory failure is due to diaphragmic weakness for patients with myasthenia gravis. For example, oropharyngeal muscle weakness can result in dysphagia leading to aspiration or upper airway obstruction.

Bedside respiratory function tests can help quantify the degree of weakness. Specifically, FVC and MIF can help guide the need for intubation. Intubation can be considered for FVC less than 15–20 cc/kg (or <1 L), MIF less than –25 cm H_2O (where approximately –50 cm H_2O is normal), or for rapid worsening. While less precise, respiratory capacity can also be assessed by asking the patient to count out loud as quickly as possible using one breath—here, counting to at least 40 is reassuring. As this patient is unable to speak in full sentences, she will likely do very poorly with this test.

Importantly, while these patients should have pulse oximetry monitoring, oxygen saturation can be falsely reassuring. In neuromuscular respiratory weakness, *hypercarbia* often occurs before hypoxemia, and so serial blood gases should be obtained.

This patient is clearly in a myasthenic crisis, which is a life-threatening complication of myasthenia gravis marked by acute exacerbation of neuromuscular weakness resulting in respiratory failure. An estimated 10–20%

of patients with myasthenia gravis may experience at least one myasthenic crisis; a similar number of patients may be first diagnosed with myasthenia gravis during a crisis.

This patient's examination is very concerning for all of the reasons just stated. Intubation at this point should be considered given her hypercarbia and poor respiratory function testing. While myasthenia gravis used to have a high mortality, ICU management with mechanical ventilation has made death from myasthenia gravis exceedingly rare.

The triggers for a myasthenic crisis are often physical stressors, such as an infection, surgery, or pregnancy; the use of a medication that can exacerbate myasthenia gravis; or the tapering of treatment.

On the differential for respiratory failure in someone with myasthenia gravis is also cholinergic crisis, which is rare but can occur in patients taking high doses of pyridostigmine, a cholinesterase inhibitor. Cholinergic crisis can be distinguished from myasthenic crisis by the presence of pupillary miosis, excessive salivation, and diarrhea, as well as muscle fasciculations and cramps.

The management of a myasthenic crisis centers on respiratory support, including elective intubation if necessary (with avoidance of neuromuscular blocking agents), emergent use of IVIg or plasma exchange, and identification and treatment of the trigger for the crisis. Plasma exchange is thought to directly remove acetylcholine receptor (AChR) antibodies from circulation, though AChR antibody titers do not correlate with disease severity or improvement. IVIg can often be provided more expeditiously than plasma exchange and does not carry the same bleeding risks. Rather, the risks associated with IVIg include thrombosis, volume overload, acute kidney injury, and anaphylaxis, especially in those who are IgA deficient, and so it is recommend to test immunoglobulin levels—but not delay treatment while waiting for these results. Plasma exchange requires the placement of a specialized central line. Potential risks include hypocalcemia, hypotension, line infection, and bleeding complications from the loss of fibrinogen, which requires daily monitoring. Plasma exchange may take effect more quickly than IVIg; however, there is limited data comparing these two treatments, and there is no clear benefit of using one over the other with regard to overall efficacy. Consult your individual hospital policy prior to IVIg or plasma exchange use.

Acutely, pyridostigmine is often held until respiratory function has improved as it can increase secretion production.

There is some controversy around the use of glucocorticoids in patients with myasthenia gravis. The initiation of high-dose glucocorticoids may result in a worsening of myasthenic symptoms in approximately half of patients, which may lead to respiratory failure in a minority of these patients. An example of this is starting high-dose steroids for a chronic obstructive pulmonary disease exacerbation in someone with myasthenia gravis, who then develops worsening myasthenic symptoms. Importantly, exacerbation of neuromuscular weakness is usually delayed, between 5 and 10 days following glucocorticoid initiation, and the effect can last for several days. It is thought that the risk of worsening once IVIg or plasma exchange has started is dramatically reduced. If a patient is intubated, then it is reasonable to initiate high-dose glucocorticoids (e.g., prednisone 60–80 mg/d). However, if the patient is experiencing worsened myasthenic symptoms but is not intubated, the risk of high-dose glucocorticoids may be too great, in which case a low dose can be tried with a very gradual up-titration. If a patient is started on steroids for an extended period of time, remember to also start supplementation for vitamin D and calcium, as well as prophylaxis for *Pneumocystis jirovecii* pneumonia and gastrointestinal ulcers.

Other immunomodulating, steroid-sparing treatments can be considered, such as azathioprine and mycophenolate mofetil, but a clinical response may take several months.

While rapid recognition and treatment has dramatically reduced mortality from myasthenic crisis, prolonged ICU admissions and ventilator days can result in significant morbidity. Providers should remain vigilant for common complications such as infection, vascular complications—including those from treatment—and cardiac complications, such as arrhythmias. Rehabilitation services should be engaged as soon as feasible.

- Neuromuscular respiratory weakness is usually associated with hypercarbia before hypoxemia.
- Triggers for a myasthenic crisis are often physical stressors, such as an infection, surgery, or pregnancy; the use of a medication that can exacerbate myasthenia gravis; or the tapering of treatment.
- While rare, consider cholinergic crisis in patients taking high doses of pyridostigmine who present with miosis, excessive salivation, diarrhea, muscle fasciculations, and/or cramps.
- In myasthenic crisis, treatment with IVIg or plasma exchange should begin emergently.

Further Reading

Gajdos P, Chevret S, Clair B, Tranchant C, Chastang C. Clinical trial of plasma exchange and high-dose intravenous immunoglobulin in myasthenia gravis. Myasthenia Gravis Clinical Study Group. *Ann Neurol.* 1997;41(6):789–796.

Gajdos P, Tranchant C, Clair B, et al. Treatment of myasthenia gravis exacerbation with intravenous immunoglobulin: a randomized double-blind clinical trial. *Arch Neurol.* 2005;62(11):1689–1693.

Gummi RR, Kukulka NA, Deroche CB, Govindarajan R. Factors associated with acute exacerbations of myasthenia gravis. *Muscle Nerve.* 2019;60(6):693–699.

Sanders DB, Wolfe GI, Benatar M, et al. International consensus guidance for management of myasthenia gravis: executive summary. *Neurology.* 2016;87(4):419–425.

29 Encephalopathy and Seizure After Transplant

A 35-year-old man with a history of hypertension and end-stage renal disease status post kidney transplant, on tacrolimus, mycophenolate, and prednisone, presents to the ED after a witnessed generalized tonic-clonic seizure. He received midazolam 5 mg IM by paramedics. In the ED, he is afebrile, blood pressure 200/100, heart rate 90. He is postictal but following simple commands, without clear focality to his exam. A nicardipine drip is started. He is loaded with fosphenytoin 20 mg/kg IV. His labs show a leukocytosis to 13 and normal electrolytes. Urine toxicology is negative. His tacrolimus level is normal. His noncontrast head CT does not reveal an acute process. He is started on vancomycin, ceftriaxone, ampicillin, and acyclovir at meningeal dosing. His lumbar puncture (LP) has a normal opening pressure, a WBC count of 2, RBC count of 5, protein 40, and glucose 81. His EEG is mildly slow and without epileptiform discharges.

What do you do now?

There are several aspects of this case that should cause concern and modify the differential diagnosis. One is that this patient recently underwent a solid organ transplant and is taking several immunosuppressant medications. He had a prodrome of feeling unwell prior to having a seizure. Last, he was markedly hypertensive on arrival. Once he is stabilized, how do you sort out what is going on?

First, his hypertension should be emergently corrected. In this patient, given his calcineurin inhibitor use, hypertension may be a sign of posterior reversible encephalopathy syndrome (PRES). PRES is a syndrome of varying severities characterized by headache, confusion, visual symptoms, and seizures with distinct neuroimaging findings often involving edema of the white matter in the posterior regions of the brain (see Figure 29.1). PRES is a misnomer as it is not always reversible, not always located in the posterior part of the brain, and is not isolated to the white matter because cortical signs and symptoms (e.g., seizure) can occur.

The underlying cause is not known but is likely due to endothelial dysfunction and cerebral autoregulation malfunction. It is associated with several conditions, including the use of immunosuppressant medications, eclampsia, and hypertension (see Box 29.1). Similar to PRES, reversible cerebral vasoconstriction syndrome (RCVS) may also be due to malfunction of cerebral autoregulation and can be triggered by vasoactive drugs; however, RCVS is characterized by evidence of arterial construction, unlike PRES. While several medications are associated with the development of PRES (Box 29.1), the development of PRES is largely idiosyncratic when it comes to duration, dose, or drug level. In addition to treating hypertension and seizure, discontinuation of the immunosuppressive therapy is usually recommended.

To formulate a differential diagnosis, it can be helpful to identify the type of transplantation (solid organ or hematopoietic cell), which organ if a solid organ transplantation was performed, and the time lapsed from the transplant itself.

Given he is immunosuppressed, he should undergo a noncontrast head CT prior to his LP. This head CT will help identify cerebral edema or any unexpected mass lesion. Solid organ transplantation recipients are at risk for infection, so an LP is crucial here if safe to perform.

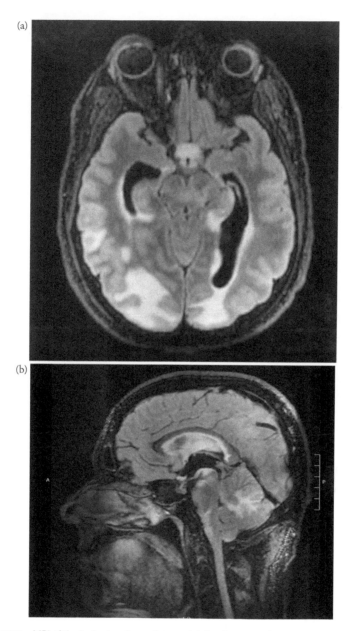

FIGURE 29.1 MRI of the brain showing parieto-occipital and posterior fossa vasogenic edema preferentially involving the white matter concerning for posterior reversible encephalopathy syndrome, shown on axial (a) and sagittal (b) views.

> **BOX 29.1** **Nonexhaustive list of medications and medical conditions associated with posterior reversible encephalopathy syndrome (PRES)**
>
> Medications
> - Calcineurin inhibitors: Tacrolimus, sirolimus, cyclosporine
> - VEGF inhibitors: Bevacizumab
> - Platinum-based agents: Cisplatin
> - Tyrosine kinase inhibitors: Sorafenib
> - Methotrexate
> - Rituximab
> - Iodine contrast
>
> Medical conditions
> - Hypertension
> - Kidney disease
> - Preeclampsia/eclampsia
> - Transplantation
> - Hematologic: Hemolytic uremic syndrome, thrombotic thrombocytopenic purpura
> - Vasculitis
> - Sepsis
> - Excessive licorice consumption (leading to hypertension)

During the first month post-transplant, these infections are often from the hospital environment or from the organ itself if the donor had an infection. After discharge, these patients remain at high risk for infection. These infections represent a wide range of pathogens, including bacteria such as *Nocardia, Listeria,* and *Mycobacterium tuberculosis*; fungi, including *Cryptococcus neoformans* and *Aspergillus* species; viruses, including the varied herpesviruses; and the parasite *Toxoplasma gondii*. Particular to this case, herpesviruses are more often associated with seizure, especially human herpesviruses 1, 2, and 6.

More than 6 months post-transplant, additional infections should be considered. JC virus targets oligodendrocytes and causes progressive multifocal leukoencephalopathy (PML), a complication with high mortality. Epstein-Barr (EBV)-associated diseases include post-transplant lymphoproliferative disorder. For this reason, it is important to check JC virus DNA PCR, cytology, and flow cytometry in CSF, in addition to obtaining an opening pressure.

MRI brain with and without contrast is warranted after the patient is stabilized. The MRI can provide more detailed information on patterns of edema or enhancement, which is important for framing the differential and trending over time.

There are several other conditions to keep in mind. In addition to chemotherapeutic medications, toxic leukoencephalopathies can occur from a variety of compounds, including amphetamines, opiates such as heroin and fentanyl, and carbon monoxide. Delayed leukoencephalopathies can be seen with radiation and anoxia. Cerebrovascular disorders may mimic these clinical and radiographic findings, including ischemic arterial and venous strokes. Malignancies in addition to lymphoma, such as carcinomatous meningitis and astrocytoma, can be considered. Immune-mediated demyelinating syndromes are more often seen in the peripheral nervous system but can also be found centrally.

In this case, PRES is a likely diagnosis. Those who develop seizures in the setting of PRES are unlikely to develop unprovoked seizures in the long-term. Antiepileptics can likely be weaned in the subsequent months provided that seizure precipitants, including hypertension, are avoided.

The prognosis of patients with PRES is overall favorable, especially if a precipitant is identified and treated. However, it is important to keep in mind that serious morbidity and even mortality can occur from cerebral edema. For example, cerebral edema can lead to hydrocephalus or other cerebrovascular complications, such as stroke. For these reasons, it is important to remain vigilant for this entity and not assume a guaranteed benign "reversible" course.

- PRES can be caused by several medications used post-transplant, especially calcineurin inhibitors such as tacrolimus and cyclosporine, and it is not always associated with a supratherapeutic drug level.
- PRES can occur at any point post-transplant, and symptoms can vary.
- Transplant recipients are at high risk for infection, and the specific risk changes over time.
- PRES may result in marked cerebral edema leading to hydrocephalus and stroke acutely, and so vigilance for these complications is paramount.

Further Reading

Datar S, Singh T, Rabinstein AA, Fugate JE, Hocker S. Long-term risk of seizures and epilepsy in patients with posterior reversible encephalopathy syndrome. *Epilepsia.* 2015;56(4):564–568.

Fugate JE, Rabinstein AA. Posterior reversible encephalopathy syndrome: clinical and radiological manifestations, pathophysiology, and outstanding questions. *Lancet Neurol.* 2015;14(9):914–925.

Kumar Y, Drumsta D, Mangla M, et al. Toxins in brain! Magnetic resonance (MR) imaging of toxic leukoencephalopathy—a pictorial essay. *Pol J Radiol.* 2017;82:311–319.

Pruitt AA, Graus F, Rosenfeld MR. Neurological complications of solid organ transplantation. *Neurohospitalist.* 2013;3(3):152–166.

30 Nonepileptic Spells

A 28-year-old woman is brought to the ED
after a series of "fits" manifested by bilateral
forceful lower extremity shaking movements
and loud verbal outbursts. A friend is with her
and states this has happened in the past "when
doctors changed her epilepsy medicine." While
you are examining her, she has another spell
with head turning from side to side, cursing,
singing, and bilateral intermittent asynchronous
leg shaking. There is no incontinence, and after
about 3 minutes the patient stops shaking,
looks at you and asks "Did I do it again?" She
is able to converse well but is agitated. Vital
signs are normal. She has several small areas
of ecchymosis. She moves all extremities well
but is a bit dysarthric. General and neurological
exams are otherwise normal.

What do you do now?

This patient's ictal behavior is decidedly inconsistent with epileptic seizures: maintenance of consciousness despite bilateral clonic limb movements, immediate return to full interactive communication after the event, singing, etc. However, before diagnosing nonepileptic spells, certain key steps must be taken. Fortunately, most medical systems have ways to share medical records electronically or at least quickly, and, for this patient, one suspects that these will be revealing of pertinent history. Metabolic screening as well as drug screening should be done, and if there are any neurological deficits, CT of the head should rule out significant intracranial pathology. Here the dysarthria may qualify as a neurologic sign so CT is probably indicated. Unfortunately, EEG is *not* particularly helpful unless another spell happens during recording. This patient apparently carries a diagnosis of epilepsy, and it is essential to control breakthrough seizures if they are occurring.

Seizures like this patient exhibits are best termed *psychogenic nonepileptic seizures* (PNES) to distinguish them from "organic" nonepileptic seizures, which refers to conditions like migraine, movement disorders, syncope, and transient ischemic attacks (TIAs) which can mimic epilepsy. PNESs are more common than was once thought, although prevalence is difficult to measure. The condition arises from psychological causes including conversion disorder, factitious disorder, and dissociative disorders. They are often seen in people who have suffered abuse or trauma. People with PNES are usually initially misdiagnosed as having epilepsy, and since it is hard to reverse that diagnosis, correct identification often takes years. Nonepileptic spells are not uncommon in patients with epilepsy (a meta-analysis of observational studies found that approximately 22% of patients with PNES had comorbid epilepsy, and approximately 12% of patients with epilepsy had PNES), making the evaluation even more challenging.

Often PNESs manifest with behavior unusual in epileptic seizures, such as asynchronous limb shaking, laughing, crying, arching of the back, and awareness of surroundings despite apparent bilateral cerebral discharges. Self-injury, like tongue biting, which is common in epileptic generalized motor seizures, is less common, as is incontinence. Triggers for PNES spells tend to be emotional or situational, and they usually occur in the presence of others. There is often a history of refractoriness to anticonvulsant medications, leading to frequent medication changes. There is also commonly a history of posttraumatic stress disorder (PTSD) and childhood sexual and physical abuse.

Diagnosis of PNES rests on video-EEG monitoring which is nearly always successful (if a spell is observed) in differentiating it from frontal lobe epilepsy and complex partial seizures which may resemble the behavioral manifestations of PNES. If this service is unavailable at your institution, it is important to refer your patient to an epilepsy center that can provide that. Once the diagnosis of PNES is made, the process of communicating this to the patient and designing a treatment program begins. This should be done in a nonjudgmental fashion, framed in a way that does not suggest that the patient is malingering, since this is usually not the case. Cognitive-behavioral therapy is reported to be helpful. Selective serotonin reuptake inhibitor (SSRI) antidepressants have been shown to be helpful in some patients as well.

When a patient with a known diagnosis of PNES is seen in the ED following a spell or series of spells, the approach can still be problematic. There are often mixed feelings on the part of the patient's medical care providers about the diagnosis, and more often than not, antiepileptic medication has been continued "just in case." This does nothing but confuse the patient and family, and it then falls to the medical team in the ED to try to make some progress toward appropriate treatment. Again, approaching the diagnosis in a nonaccusatory way is essential in order to make any real progress. Psychiatric consultation should be sought, and obtaining previous video-EEG data can be very useful as well. It is important to avoid repetition of diagnostic testing and escalation of antiepileptic medication.

KEY POINTS TO REMEMBER

- The diagnosis of PNES is challenging, and patients may be misdiagnosed with epilepsy for years.
- Clues to the diagnosis of PNES can be found in the ictal presentation, as well as in the patient's description of triggers.
- Video-EEG monitoring is generally successful in distinguishing PNES from epilepsy.
- Communicating the diagnosis to the patient must be done in a clear and consistent but nonaccusatory way.

Further Reading

Avbersek A, Sisodiya S. Does the primary literature provide support for clinical signs used to distinguish psychogenic nonepileptic seizures from epileptic seizures? *J Neurol Neurosurg Psychiatry* 2010;81:719–725.

Brown RJ, Reuber M. Towards an integrative theory of psychogenic non-epileptic seizures (PNES). *Clin Psychol Rev.* 2016;47:55–70.

Carlson P, Perry KN. Psychological interventions for psychogenic non-epileptic seizures: a meta-analysis. *Seizure.* 2017;45:142–150.

Carton S, Thompson PJ, Duncan JS. Non-epileptic seizures: patients' understanding and reaction to the diagnosis and impact on outcome. *Seizure.* 2003;12(5):287–294.

Kutlubaev MA, Xu Y, Hackett ML, Stone J. Dual diagnosis of epilepsy and psychogenic nonepileptic seizures: systematic review and meta-analysis of frequency, correlates, and outcomes. *Epilepsy Behav.* 2018;89:70–78.

LaFrance WC Jr, Baird GL, et al. Multicenter pilot treatment trial for psychogenic nonepileptic seizures: a randomized clinical trial. *JAMA Psychiatry.* 2014;71(9):997–1005.

Reuber M, Fernandez G, Bauer J, et al. Diagnostic delay in psychogenic nonepileptic seizures. *Neurology.* 2002;58(3):493–495.

31 Migraine in a Pregnant Patient

A 26-week pregnant 30-year-old woman with a long history of migraines is seen in the ED with 2 days of unrelenting diffuse severe headache pain that came on gradually. The accompanying nausea has led to incessant vomiting—"there is nothing left to throw up" she tells the ED physician. She also describes lightheadedness and blurred vision but no other neurological symptoms. She has not had auras. Her examination is normal, although she is clearly fatigued. She is taking only perinatal vitamins.

What do you do now?

Many women with migraine experience improvement and even remission in their headaches during pregnancy by the time of their second trimester. This tends to be even more likely in women with menstrually related migraine attacks. But there are still many women who experience the opposite trend, with recurring, disabling head pain and nausea during pregnancy. The first decision in this type of case, of course, is how seriously to workup the changes in her migraine symptoms, primarily, the intensity of pain and nausea. Gestational hypertension and preeclampsia must be ruled out, of course. Of note, there is some evidence that eclampsia occurs more often and earlier in pregnancy in women with migraine. Elevated blood pressure, proteinuria, and elevated hepatic enzymes (seen in HELLP syndrome along with anemia and thrombocytopenia) are diagnostic. Meningitis or encephalitis are considered with meningismus, altered mental state, fever, or leukocytosis. Without focal neurological deficits, an intracranial mass, inflammatory, or infectious process is unlikely. Cerebral venous thrombosis and idiopathic intracranial hypertension (IIH) are, however, possible, and if clinical suspicion is high or if there are even subtle neurological findings on exam (optic disc swelling, dysconjugate gaze, mild mental status alteration, etc.), a head MRI, MR venogram, and lumbar puncture (LP) would be indicated. The poorly understood syndrome of "postpartum angiopathy," also known as the *reversible cerebral vasoconstriction syndrome* (RCVS), could be possible here, which would require imaging of the cerebral vessels and can be accomplished with CT angiogram or MR angiogram time-of-flight, as gadolinium should be avoided during pregnancy. However, RCVS tends to be limited to the puerperium or late pregnancy and tends to include recurrent thunderclap (sudden) headaches and sometimes focal neurological deficits, none of which is present in this case. Pituitary hemorrhage tends to present with sudden headache and visual acuity and field deficits, but history can be vague, and, contrary to previous belief, this is not necessarily limited to the peripartum period (a case series and literature review by Grandmaison in 2015 found the median gestational age was in fact 24 weeks). To rule this out, CT or MRI might be best.

Once secondary causes of acute severe headache are excluded, status migrainosus is the most likely diagnosis here and constitutes an urgent management need. If vomiting has led to dehydration, intravenous rehydration must be done, ideally with a bolus of normal saline to avoid fetal compromise. While neuroleptic antinauseants are not known to be safe in pregnancy, it is common practice to use metoclopramide 10 mg, promethazine 25 mg, or prochlorperazine 10 mg intravenously. These have the added benefit of reducing headache pain as well as nausea in many cases. This class of medication can, of course, lead to dystonia or akathisia, appearing generally within minutes after administration. Infusing diphenhydramine (generally considered safe in pregnancy) 25 mg IV at least 15 minutes prior to antinauseant use can help to prevent the dystonia, although it is less effective in akathisa.

Even without preeclampsia, magnesium infusion can be very helpful as magnesium sulfate at a dose of 1 g slow IV push or dissolved in normal saline. However, magnesium should be used sparingly as it may increase the risk of fetal osteopenia. On occasion greater occipital nerve blocks, generally done bilaterally, can be very helpful for acute migraine, and trigger point injections can be useful as well, although evidence is lacking for these interventions. Massage and ice application to the head and neck can be surprisingly helpful, and, after nausea is controlled, these may suffice along with rest. But more intensive pharmacotherapy is often needed.

Medication choices in pregnancy are limited. There are some data about drug safety in pregnancy, but sources of information differ. The US Food and Drug Administration (FDA) has in the past provided a listing of relative safety, using five categories A, B, C, D, and X (see Box 31.1). Unfortunately, very few drugs are in the "safer" categories (A and B) and many drugs are not rated. Another rating system, the Teratogen Information Service (TERIS) of the University of Washington also provides risk categories for many drugs from "no risk" to "high risk." Unfortunately, many drugs are rated "undetermined" or "unlikely." And the FDA and TERIS ratings often do not concur.

Acetaminophen is in the FDA category B, and, used intravenously in a dose of 1,000 mg, it can be surprisingly effective even in cases where oral acetaminophen has been ineffective. Non-steroidal anti-inflammatory medications are probably best avoided as there is some evidence of fetal risk in the first and third trimesters. The use of parenteral opioids is controversial. The only opioids which are in category B are oxycodone, butorphanol, meperidine, and morphine. Morphine is preferred; it has been observed, however, that after responding to opioid medication, migraine tends to recur (see Table 31.1 and Box 31.2).

Triptans, particularly sumatriptan, seem to be safe during pregnancy based on pregnancy registry data, although it is not known with certainty, and all are category C. Most headache specialists advocate occasional use of sumatriptan, and in the 6 mg subcutaneous form it can be highly effective even in status migrainosus. Ergots, including ergotamine and dihydroergotamine are Category X, due to their effects on implantation of the embryo, uterine blood flow, and fetal development as well as their tendency to produce uterine contractions.

Of the antiemetics, metoclopramide is in category B; prochlorperazine and promethazine are in category C, but all have been used when nausea and vomiting lead to dehydration and/or metabolic imbalances in pregnant women.

Corticosteroid use in pregnancy has been linked to premature birth and low birth weight, and corticosteroids are Category C. In the ED setting,

TABLE 31.1 **Selected medications for acute migraine commonly used in pregnancy**

Medication	FDA category	TERIS risk rating
Acetaminophen	B (oral), C (IV)	No risk
Ibuprofen	B (D in 3rd trimester)	Minimal
Naproxen	B (D in 3rd trimester)	Undetermined
Ketorolac	D	
Hydromorphone	C	
Morphine	C	
Magnesium sulfate IV	B (limited to 5 days to avoid fetal osteopenia)	Unlikely
Metoclopramide	B	Unlikely
Prednisone	C in 1st trimester; less clear in 2nd/3rd trimesters	Minimal
Promethazine	C	None
Prochlorperazine	C	None
Chlorpromazine	C	None

methylprednisolone 1 g IV can eventually help break a long-lasting migraine and help to prevent recurrence.

After the headache is controlled, it is worth thinking about prophylaxis in order to prevent recurrence. Agents such as beta blockers, calcium channel blockers, and cyclic antidepressants are all Category C agents (except for atenolol which is Category D) and may not even be that effective at preventing migraine during pregnancy. Topiramate is in Category D. A number of medications used to treat migraine can alter folate metabolism so supplementing with 0.4 mg/d folate is advisable when using daily medications.

A stepwise approach to the pregnant patient with acute severe headache

1. Vital signs, IV hydration, thorough general and neurological exam including careful mental status and funduscopic exam; CBC, complete chemistry panel, urinalysis including toxic screen. Try to create a quiet, dark environment, use cold application and massage if possible.

2. If HA is new to patient, recent trauma, vital signs are abnormal, neurological exam is in any way abnormal (or cannot be completed) or meningismus is present, rule out intracranial hemorrhage, intracranial hypertension, cerebral venous thrombosis, infection, and RCVS, with all of the appropriate following testing: CT or MRI (and perhaps CT or MR angiography), and lumbar puncture.

3. If workup complete and reassuring, assume migraine, and treat with diphenhydramine 25 mg IV followed by metoclopramide 10 mg IV.

4. Magnesium sulfate 1 g to be repeated up to 3 more times every 30 min, with cardiac monitoring.

5. Consider IV acetaminophen 1,000 mg IV, sumatriptan 6 mg subcutaneously, or morphine 1–2 mg IV which can be repeated.

6. Methylprednisolone 1 g IV.

KEY POINTS TO REMEMBER

- While migraines improve during pregnancy for most women, there are many cases of the opposite, sometimes accompanied by severe nausea and vomiting.
- Suspicion for secondary cause of headaches such as cerebral venous thrombosis, RCVS, and hemorrhage should be high with any change in headache pattern, although most headaches will be benign.

- Nonpharmacological therapy such as massage, local application of cold, and rest in a quiet dark place can help, particularly after nausea and dehydration are corrected.
- Pharmaceutical treatment of pain is indicated in severe cases and can include parenteral magnesium, acetaminophen, and opioids used cautiously.

Further Reading

Ayer R, Schmutz T, Guechi Y, Ribordy V. Headaches in pregnancy: management in the emergency department. *Revue medicale suisse*. 2018;14:1405–1407.

Briggs GB, Freeman RK, Towers CV, Forinash AB. *Drugs in Pregnancy and Lactation: A Reference Guide to Fetal and Neonatal Risk* (11th ed.). New York: Lippincott Williams & Wilkins; 2017.

Sandoe CH, Lay C. Secondary headaches during pregnancy: when to worry. *Curr NeurolNeurosci Rep*. 2019;19(6):27.

Pediatric Dilemmas

32 Acute Migraine in a Child

A 25 kg 9-year-old boy with recurrent migraine
headaches awoke with a particularly severe
headache this morning. He has been vomiting
all morning and has been unresponsive to
oral analgesics and antiemetics. In the ED, IV
ketorolac has been only minimally helpful.
IV prochlorperazine has helped the nausea,
but severe headache persists. General and
neurological exams are normal. CT has not been
done in order to avoid exposure to radiation.

What do you do now?

This boy seems to have a typical case of migraine, which is not un-common (before puberty, male and female prevalence of migraine is roughly equal), but the intense severity is unusual. The unremitting vomiting and intractability of the pain is also a bit unusual but not unheard of. A thorough neurological examination, including comprehensive mental status exam, should be performed to make sure there really is no focal deficit. If this is normal, then a CT scan is probably not necessary. An MRI may be worthwhile at some point to exclude an intracranial mass, arteriovenous malformation, or congenital cranial malformations. The general examination should focus on evidence of trauma, accidental or inflicted, as well as any signs of infection or general medical issues. Meningismus should be carefully looked for. It is important to check basic metabolic function regarding electrolyte balance (especially given the persistent vomiting), glucose level, blood counts, and hepatic and renal function. Ruling out infection is crucial since urinary, pulmonary, ear, and other infections can induce severe migraine.

A good first step in treating this boy is to make sure to replace lost fluids intravenously. This will provide the added benefit of IV access for potentially useful pain- and nausea-relieving medications. Other than the neuroleptic/antiemetics, medications that might be useful for the nausea include ondansetron and hydroxyzine. Ondansetron is available as a sublingual 4 mg or 8 mg wafer that children often tolerate well, although it is not known to be entirely safe in this patient's age group. The dose is in the 0.15 mg/kg range, so 4 mg would be just right. Hydroxyzine is an antihistaminic which has both antiemetic and analgesic, as well as anxiolytic properties, and it can be given orally or intravenously in a dosage of approximately 0.25–0.5 mg/kg.

Other than acetaminophen and ibuprofen, there is very little evidence of safety or efficacy of any acute antimigraine medication. Sumatriptan and rizatriptan oral tablets and zolmitriptan nasal spray have been studied in children and seem to be safe and effective. Adverse effects are generally mild but can include taste disturbance, nasal congestion, dizziness, fatigue, low energy, nausea, or vomiting. Subcutaneous sumatriptan has been used successfully in adolescents and children, and there are now lower dose sumatriptan cartridges—3 mg and 4 mg—which would be appropriate for larger children and adolescents. While ergots are not known to be safe in children, dihydroergotamine (DHE) in a dose of approximately 0.25 mg IV for preteens and 0.5–1.0 mg for teens has been used successfully. An antinauseant should be used along with DHE since it can be quite nauseating.

Most children and adolescents will find that the migraine resolves after sleep. Most of the antinauseants have some soporific effects, which can be an added benefit. Good choices include promethazine 0.5–1 mg/kg orally or rectally, or prochlorperazine 0.15 mg/kg in parenteral, rectal, or oral forms. It is important to remember that dyskinesia can occur; pretreatment with diphenhydramine tends to prevent this. Akathisia is also possible and tends to respond to low doses of parenteral benzodiazepines.

Hydroxyzine likewise has a sedative and analgesic effect; it can be useful in a dose of 0.5–1 mg/kg in oral or parenteral routes. In rare cases, when none of these seems to work, deeper sedation and analgesia may be needed, which can be achieved with barbiturates or opioids. If this approach is necessary, it should probably be done on an inpatient basis so that the patient can be observed carefully.

Most children with severe migraine are to some extent scared or nervous about the intensity of the acute experiences. A quiet, dark room is essential for acute treatment to be most effective. Reassurance is essential. More formal counseling can help, and this also opens the door for subsequent family counseling that could help to reduce triggers and defuse some of the drama for all family members that can escalate during the acute attacks. Medication overuse must be screened for. If headaches are frequent, lead to frequent ED visits, or lead to missed social or family events, the use of preventive measures must be considered—and probably a referral to a pediatric neurologist/headache specialist is warranted.

KEY POINTS TO REMEMBER

- With severe migraine in a child, secondary causes must be ruled out including neurological infections, intracranial mass, and systemic metabolic or infectious disease.
- There is little evidence to aid in choosing agents for acute migraine treatment in children.

- Triptans can be very effective, as can antinauseants and sedatives.
- Most children with severe recurrent migraine headaches find them to be emotionally stressful and may benefit from counseling.

Further Reading

Lewis D, Ashwal S, Hershey A, Hirtz D, Yonker M, Silberstein S. Pharamacological treatment of migraine headache in children and adolescents: Report of the American Academy of Neurology Quality Standards Subcommittee and the Practice Committee of the Child Neurology Society. *Neurology.* 2004;63:2215–2224.

Linder SL. Subcutaneous sumatriptan in the clinical setting: the first 50 consecutive patients with acute migraine in a pediatric neurology office practice. *Headache.* 1996;36(7):419–422.

Oskoui M, Pringsheim T, Holler-Managan Y, et al. Practice guideline update summary: Acute treatment of migraine in children and adolescents: report of the Guideline Development, Dissemination, and Implementation Subcommittee of the American Academy of Neurology and the American Headache Society. *Neurology.* 2019;93(11):487–499.

Patniyot IR, Gelfand AA. Acute treatment therapies for pediatric migraine: a qualitative systematic review. *Headache.* 2016;56(1):49–70.

Richer LP, Laycock K, Millar K, et al. Treatment of children with migraine in emergency departments: national practice variation study. *Pediatrics.* 2010;126:e150–e155.

33 Febrile Seizure

A 3-year-old girl is brought to the ED after having
a generalized seizure in her sleep witnessed by
her mother who is a nurse. She describes diffuse
body stiffening, followed by generalized limb
shaking. The mother relates that her daughter
seemed to stop breathing and looked "cyanotic."
The seizure lasted approximately 15 minutes
and was followed by mild somnolence which
has persisted now for 1 hour. She recently had
a gastrointestinal viral syndrome with diarrhea
and vomiting, accompanied by fever up to 103°F,
but she has only had "at most" a mild fever
over the past 12 hours, according to the mother.
Now rectal temperature is 100.5°F, the child is
breathing regularly at 12 breaths per minute,
and pulse is 82. She is arousable but sleepy.
She moves all extremities, and there are normal
reflexes.

What do you do now?

Benign febrile seizures generally occur in children between 3 months and 5 years of age. The mechanism is unknown, but predisposing genetic factors have been postulated because different genetic strains in animal models have required different temperature thresholds for seizure production. Fever generally needs to be above 102°F in children. The annual incidence is probably between 5% and 10%. These seizures are usually single, generalized, and last less than 15 minutes. The child should be otherwise neurologically healthy and without neurological abnormality by examination or by developmental history. If there is any focality to the seizure, if it is prolonged, or if there are any focal neurological findings on exam, this does not qualify as a "simple febrile seizure" (see Box 33.1).

In this case there are a couple of features that are a bit unsettling. First, the seizure was rather prolonged. Fifteen minutes is still within the "simple" febrile seizure window, but it was at the upper limit. The mother should be a good historian as she is a nurse, but parents may overestimate the duration of seizures, so the actual duration may have been shorter. This child may or may not have been febrile at the time, although this is not clear. But most importantly, she is not returning to completely normal consciousness. This could be explained, however, by the time of night, falling in the middle of her normal sleep cycle. The cyanosis is actually not that uncommon, with some children seemingly becoming apneic for a short time.

BOX 33.1 **Features of "simple" febrile seizures**

Febrile at the time of the seizure
Single seizure
Age between 3 months and 5 years
Generalized without evidence of focality
Duration less than 15 minutes
Normal neurological exam
Normal developmental history

The most important question to ask is whether this seizure could be due to meningitis or encephalitis. Lumbar puncture (LP), while not usually necessary for simple febrile seizures, would not be a bad idea here. There is scant risk of causing brain herniation with a nonfocal neurological exam, but CT of the head could be done to rule out a mass. Since serum glucose will be drawn to compare with CSF glucose, adding electrolytes, calcium, and perhaps magnesium and a CBC is probably worth doing even though this is generally not necessary in patients with benign febrile seizures. LP is particularly worthwhile in infants between 6 and 12 months of age who present with a seizure and fever who have not received the usual *Haemophilus influenzae* or *Streptococcus pneumoniae* immunizations.

Once CNS infection is ruled out, it might be worthwhile searching further for a structural cause for the seizure. However, when febrile seizures do not recur, and if the patient fully awakens with no residual deficits, MRI scanning of the brain is not considered necessary. EEG might provide some evidence of an epileptic focus in a few patients with febrile seizures, but it is probably not indicated for this patient. If she awakens fully, CSF is normal, and no abnormalities are seen on the basic blood testing, there is also no reason to admit her to the hospital.

Finally, the questions of future seizure risk and the need for prophylactic treatment generally arises. Patients with simple febrile seizures have only a slightly higher risk of recurrent seizures (unless they again occur during a fever in the right age range) than any other person. Children with "complex febrile seizures" (not fulfilling the requirements for simple febrile seizures) are much more likely to have epilepsy later, probably in the 80% range. Since this patient essentially falls within the benign febrile seizure group, she should not have a significantly increased risk of seizure occurrence. Prophylaxis with antiepileptic medication is generally not recommended for children who have single febrile seizures since the benefit is low and there are significant side effects to all antiepileptic medications, particularly cognitive slowing. If the parent's concern is high, EEG can be helpful in identifying any potential seizure focus which might suggest prophylactic treatment.

- Simple febrile seizures generally do not require lab investigation.
- If there is any suspicion of meningitis or encephalitis, LP should be strongly considered.
- Focal seizure activity, prolonged duration of the seizure (>15 minutes), multiple seizures, older age (>5 years old), or abnormal neurological exam should prompt a more careful investigation.
- Prophylaxis is not indicated for single simple febrile seizures.

Further Reading

American Academy of Pediatrics Subcommittee on Febrile Seizures. Febrile seizures: guideline for the neurodiagnostic evaluation of the child with a simple febrile seizure: clinical practice guideline. *Pediatrics.* 2011;127:389–394.

Natsume J, Hamano SI, Iyoda K, et al. New guidelines for management of febrile seizures in Japan. *Brain Dev.* 2017;39(1):2–9.

Smith DK, Sadler KP, Benedum M. Febrile seizures: risks, evaluation, and prognosis. *Am Fam Phys.* 2019;99(7):445–450.

34 Acute Ataxia in a Child

A 7-year-old girl is brought to the ER by her mother because of gait difficulty. She had been well until yesterday, when she began stumbling while walking; when she tried to play soccer with her friend, she kept falling. She has no other symptoms and general exam is normal with blood pressure 90/60, pulse regular at 76, respirations 14, and temperature of 98°F. Birth and past medical history are unremarkable, and there is no family history of neurological disease. On neurological exam, mental status is intact. Cranial nerves are normal except for sustained, direction-changing horizontal nystagmus and mild dysarthria that the mother and child also appreciate. Motor tone and strength are intact, as is sensation. Reflexes are present and symmetrical. She has difficulty with gait, truncal instability, and incoordination of limbs. CT of the head is entirely normal.

What do you do now?

The examination is primarily concerning for a process affecting the cerebellum and is notable for both axial and appendicular ataxia. Differential diagnosis of the acute cerebellar syndrome in children (Box 34.1) includes structural lesions and infectious or postinfectious etiologies, as well as toxic and metabolic causes.

Structural causes include tumors such as cerebellar astrocytoma or medulloblastoma, ischemic stroke (such as secondary to a vertebral artery dissection), or hemorrhage. For this reason, it is important to inquire about recent head or neck trauma. CT scan of the head should rule most of these, but MRI with contrast is the preferred imaging test. Vessel imaging of the

---

BOX 34.1   **Causes of acute childhood ataxia**

Structural
    Brain tumor
    Head trauma
    Cerebellar ischemic stroke
    Cerebellar hemorrhagic stroke
    Vertebrobasilar dissection
    Cerebellar abscess
Infectious
    Meningitis or encephalitis
    Cerebellar abscess
    Labyrinthitis
Postinfectious or autoimmune
    Acute cerebellar ataxia syndrome
    Miller Fisher syndrome
    Acute disseminated encephalomyelitis
    Opsoclonus/myoclonus syndrome
Toxic
    Alcohol
    Other drugs of abuse
    Antiepileptic toxicity, especially phenytoin
Metabolic
    Inborn error of metabolism

head and neck should be obtained if a vascular cause is likely. A posterior fossa mass seems unlikely in this case given the acute nature of this presentation, but a stroke or a mass that bleeds can definitely present acutely.

An abscess is an infectious lesion that can present acutely. Meningitis and encephalitis must also be considered as these are associated with high morbidity and mortality, and so CSF should be obtained if there is concern for infection. Cerebellar inflammation (cerebellitis) from an infectious cause includes *Listeria monocytogenes*, Lyme disease, Epstein-Barr virus, varicella zoster virus and Coxsackie virus. Treatment and recovery depend on the isolated pathogen. Acute disseminated encephalomyelitis (ADEM) is a rare cause of ataxia that can also occur following an infection. In addition to cerebellar ataxia, ADEM may also be associated with multifocal neurological deficits, seizures, or altered mental status. MRI in ADEM should be abnormal, and CSF will often have a pleocytosis and elevated protein.

It is important to keep in mind that cerebellar edema or a space-occupying lesion in the posterior fossa is a neurologic emergency. Depending on the cause, treatment may include steroids and/or surgical decompression. An external ventricular drain (EVD) must be carefully considered because a supratentorial EVD placement without infratentorial decompression can result in upward herniation.

Accidental ingestion of medication such as anticonvulsants can lead to ataxia, and some detective work along these lines might be fruitful. Toxins such as ethanol or illicit drugs can also lead to cerebellar dysfunction and must be excluded with toxicology studies. While this patient does not have the typical back pain and lower extremity weakness seen in spinal cord lesions like discitis, myelopathy with sensory and/or motor dysfunction should be kept in mind as a cause of ataxia, though this would not explain the bulbar symptoms.

Miller Fisher syndrome, a variant of Guillain-Barré syndrome, may present with acute cerebellar symptoms and signs but is often accompanied by hyporeflexia and ophthalmoplegia. Opsoclonus/myoclonus syndrome is another possibility, also known as "dancing eyes-dancing feet." This is a paraneoplastic autoimmune disorder seen in children with neuroblastoma and manifests as migratory myoclonic jerks as dramatic jumping eye movements (opsoclonus) and ataxia. This patient did have mild nystagmus but did not have the prerequisite opsoclonic movements or myoclonic jerks. Acute labyrinthitis can lead to the appearance of ataxia, and children might not be able to explain that their balance/gait difficulties stem from vertigo rather than imbalance. However, nausea is usually preeminent, and children are generally quite distressed with vertigo. Posttraumatic vertigo may also be considered, and so inquiring about recent head trauma, even mild, can be helpful.

When other more ominous possibilities are ruled out, acute cerebellar ataxia syndrome, which is largely postinfectious, is likely. This has been observed following a number of infections including varicella, Epstein-Barr virus, mycoplasma, enterovirus, roseola, rubeola, and parvovirus. The syndrome is generally seen in children between 2 and 7 years old but has been reported in older children and adults. It accounts for approximately 40–50% of the cases of acute ataxia in children. The mechanism is presumably immune-mediated cerebellar inflammation, and there have also been cases of acute ataxia in children who have recently had vaccinations. Other than truncal and limb ataxia with gait difficulty, there are generally no other accompanying symptoms. Some children have nystagmus, as did this child.

While often a benign, monophasic illness, it is important to remember that postinfectious cerebellitis can be complicated by significant cerebellar edema. For this reason, brain imaging should be pursued in any ataxic patient, and lumbar puncture (LP) should also be considered, especially if the patient also presents with altered mental status, asymmetric or progressive neurologic deficits, or headache.

KEY POINTS TO REMEMBER

- Acute childhood ataxia is often due to a benign self-limited postinfectious condition.
- Accurate history is important to assure that the ataxia is acute rather than gradually progressive and to rule out accidental ingestions and accompanying symptoms.
- Workup of acute ataxia in a child should include head CT or MRI. LP should be performed if there is concern for an infectious or inflammatory cause.

Further Reading

Salas, AA, Nava, A. Acute cerebellar ataxia in childhood: initial approach in the emergency department. *Emerg Med J.* 2010;27:956–957.

Van der Maas, NAT, Vermeer-de Bondt, PE, de Melker, H, Kemmeren, JM. Acute cerebellar ataxia in the Netherlands: a study on the association with vaccinations and varicella zoster infection *Vaccine.* 2009;27:1970–1973.

35 Concussion in an Adolescent

A 16-year-old boy is brought to the ED by his soccer coach after an injury during practice 2 hours ago. His head collided with the shoulder of another player, and the patient was knocked to the ground. He may have had a brief loss of consciousness but was able to get up and walk off the field on his own. He was seen to "wander around" the sidelines for the next 30 minutes. General exam including vital signs is normal, although there seems to be some ecchymosis and tenderness in the left frontotemporal scalp. CT of the brain is negative. Mental status exam is remarkable for some disorientation to date and time, and poor memory for recent events. His speech seems a bit slow, but language is otherwise normal. Cranial nerves, motor tone and strength, sensation, coordination and balance are all intact. The coach wants to know if it is "OK if he plays in the championship game tomorrow?"

What do you do now?

Concussion, now also known as "mild traumatic brain injury (mTBI)" is defined as a change in neuropsychiatric function after a blow to the head. There need not be a loss of consciousness. Clearly there is a spectrum of severity to acute post-head injury syndromes, and many researchers have attempted to classify these by analyzing symptoms and signs following injury in an effort to plan best treatment and predict recovery for each patient. But this has proved difficult, perhaps because of a large range of individual reactions to brain injury. One conclusion seems clear: even mild head injuries can lead to lasting sequelae in some people.

It is important to rule out epidural, subdural, and intracerebral hemorrhage in these patients as soon as possible (see Figure 35.1). CT is very sensitive and, as in the presenting case, usually helps to definitively rule these out. The tenderness over this boy's frontotemporal scalp is unsettling because it is the general vicinity of the middle meningeal artery, which is the most common artery to cause epidural hematoma when lacerated by fractured skull components. Interestingly, epidural hematomas will often present with the classic pattern of loss of consciousness, lucid interval, and then progressive deterioration, so this history is crucial to obtain. Skull fractures can be missed but must be discovered as they can also lead to the very serious sequelae of CNS infection, delayed bleeding, and cranial nerve damage. Raccoon eyes (periorbital ecchymosis), Battle's sign (ecchymosis over the mastoid), otorrhea, and rhinorrhea are suggestive signs of basal skull fracture, but careful review of inferior views on the head CT is also imperative. And careful assessment of the neurological exam with special attention to the cranial nerves is essential.

In patients with normal head CT scans, all is still not worry-free. Petecchial hemorrhaging might have occurred, generally in anterior frontal and/or anterior temporal regions due to the net result of force vectors resulting from trauma, and this can progress. When these small areas of bleeding occur, often not apparent on initial CT scanning, they can later coalesce and become true cerebral contusions, sometimes 24–48 hours later. These can then lead to increased intracranial pressure and focal neurological deficits. Thus, repeating CT scans if patients seem to regress, or even if they do not clearly recover to their baseline, makes sense, as do a screening blood count and bleeding parameters in patients who have sustained head injury.

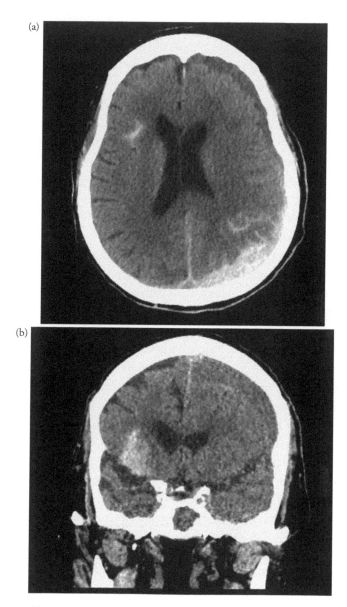

FIGURE 35.1 Noncontrast CT of the head of a child following head trauma (a) axial view revealing multicompartment intracranial parenchymal hemorrhages and left holohemispheric subdural hematoma with midline shift, (b) Coronal view showing right frontal parenchymal hemorrhage and left subdural hematoma.

What can be done in the acute period to hasten recovery in cases of mTBI like this one? This area is hotly debated, and while many feel that physical and mental rest for some time after injury is essential, there is evidence that this does not provide benefit. There is at this point no evidence that medication or supplements offer any protection or help.

So, assuming that all of the important workup is negative, can this young man return to play tomorrow? A consensus statement published by the *British Journal of Sports Medicine* suggests that any athlete, 18 and under, who may have sustained a concussion during sports should not be allowed to return to activity the same day. In the past this group believed that it was appropriate for the athlete to return to activity if cleared by a doctor or certified athletic trainer. The change came since it became clear that there is no way to make an immediate determination of safety. The American Academy of Neurology published a position statement in 2013 stating that (1) athletes who have had a concussion of any severity be immediately removed from participation and (2) the concussed athlete *not* return to participation until cleared by a physician with training in sports concussion. Numerous researchers have attempted to refine and direct treatment, return to play guidelines, and prognosis based on symptoms and signs in patients following concussion, such as amnesia, headache, cognitive dysfunction, balance, etc., but unfortunately these all tend to occur to some degree and seem not be good predictors of future status. For example, virtually all concussed patients develop some retro- and anterograde amnesia, much of which resolves.

A number of patients will have persistent symptoms of the "postconcussive syndrome" which can last for months or even indefinitely, including headaches, dizziness, cognitive difficulties, sleep abnormalities, fatigue, and mood disturbances. These symptoms can occur either singly or as the full syndrome and can become disabling, leading to falling behind in school and to a great deal of emotional suffering. The cause(s) of these symptoms is not entirely clear, but this is being actively investigated, in large part due to the growing numbers of returning soldiers concussed in combat as well as in noncombat areas and the alarming reports of many athletes suffering long-term effects of repeated concussions. It is now clear that chronic traumatic encephalopathy (CTE) is not uncommon after multiple head injuries, even when there seems to have been reasonably good recovery from each of them.

And it takes little imagination to suspect that a single identified concussion may actually be the latest in a series.

One tool for understanding the results of TBI is diffusion tensor imaging (DTI), which is being used to assess white matter changes, thought by many to bear the brunt of force vectors delivered to the head. This and other imaging test results are also being correlated with neuropsychiatric testing before and after the athletic season in an attempt to quantify cognitive changes. Of course, the athletes who are being tested are often canny enough to know that if they show a significant drop in cognition over the season, their coach may be reluctant to play them next year. As a result, preseason test scores can be artificially low.

At any rate, this patient certainly cannot go back to the field today. He may even need to be admitted to the hospital for careful observation and, if he does not improve, perhaps a repeat CT scan of the head to ensure that contusions have not formed. If he is entirely back to normal tomorrow, the question about return to play will be a difficult one. One important thing to always consider is that a second head injury can be devastating, for unclear reasons, so to be safe, most would consider this patient to be best served by some time off contact sports. How long is not clear.

KEY POINTS TO REMEMBER

· Concussion is defined as a change in neuropsychiatric function after a blow to the head, with or without loss of consciousness.
· Severe sequelae of head injury, such as epidural, subdural, and intracerebral hematomata must be ruled out acutely.
· Cerebral contusions can be delayed and should be investigated if the patient does not improve or regresses.
· There is consensus that return to the field the same day after a sports injury is contraindicated, but the benefit of longer rest times is not clear.

Further Reading
Giza CC, Kutcher JS, Ashwal S, et al. Summary of evidence-based guideline update: evaluation and management of concussion in sports: report of the

Guideline Development Subcommittee of the American Academy of Neurology. *Neurology.* 2013;80(24):2250–2257.

Gupta A, Summerville G, Senter C. Treatment of acute sports-related concussion. *Curr Rev Musculoskel Med.* 2019;12(2):117–123.

McCrea MA, Nelson LD, Guskiewicz K. Diagnosis and management of acute concussion. *Phys Med Rehabil Clin.* 2017;28(2):271–286.

McCerory, P, Meeuwisse, W, Johnston, K, Dvorak, J, Aubry, M, Molloy, M, Cantu, R. Consensus statement on concussion in sport: the 3rd International Conference on Concussion in Sport. *Br J Sports Med.* 2009;43(Suppl I):i76–i84.

Willer BS, Haider MN, Bezherano I, Wilber CG, Mannix R, Kozlowski K, Leddy JJ. Comparison of rest to aerobic exercise and placebo-like treatment of acute sport-related concussion in male and female adolescents. *Arch Phys Med Rehabil.* 2019;100(12):2267–2275.

36 Acute Stroke in an Adolescent

A 17-year-old girl with a history of depression and prior suicide attempts is brought in by parents for progressively worsening confusion. Her parents discovered her that morning, when they returned from a weekend trip, lying on her right side on a hard linoleum floor with an empty Benadryl container nearby. Her blood pressure is 155/80, heart rate 110 and regular, her breaths are 20 breaths per minute and shallow. Her ECG shows a QTc 520. In the ED you notice that her alertness waxes and wanes, speech is garbled. Her pupils are dilated and respond symmetrically to light, and she has blink to threat present bilaterally. You notice she seems to be moving her right arm and leg less than her left side. You wonder if she may have had a stroke, but your colleague says you are overreacting, that she just needs to be treated for a drug overdose.

What do you do now?

While this patient is exhibiting signs of drug toxicity, there are also focal signs on her exam that are concerning for stroke (e.g., aphasia, right-sided weakness). Stroke can occur in children and adolescents for the same major reasons that adults succumb: athero-thrombosis and embolism. And, although the risks are much lower, stroke in adolescence is not rare and can occur from a variety of reasons, including hematologic, cardiac, vascular (both noninflammatory and inflammatory), and genetic etiologies.

A major cause of stroke in children and adolescents is sickle cell disease due to spontaneous thrombosis, which can occur in any cerebral vessel. Sickle trait does not lead to an increased risk of stroke. A number of coagulopathies can lead to stroke at young ages including protein C and S deficiencies, factor V-Leiden deficiency, and others. Leukemia can also lead to stroke, both from the hypercoagulable state of cancer and from the abnormal increase of cells in the blood vessels. Neuroblastoma, other childhood neoplasms, and inflammatory states such as inflammatory bowel disease, can also cause hypercoagulability which can predispose to arterial or venous thrombosis.

Congenital heart disease is an important risk factor for stroke in childhood. Endocarditis and rheumatic heart disease can increase the risk of clot formation leading to arterial stroke. A patent foramen ovale (PFO) can lead to paradoxical embolic events. Those who undergo cardiac surgery are also at risk of perioperative stroke.

Several noninflammatory vasculopathies may cause pediatric stroke. Moyamoya disease is a progressive steno-occlusive arteriopathy that affects the anterior circulation. Arterial dissection of the carotid or vertebral arteries can occur spontaneously or secondary to trauma or connective tissue disease. Inflammatory vascular diseases can also lead to stroke, including primary CNS vasculitis, Takayasu's arteritis, polyarteritis nodosa, and other rheumatologic diseases. Infectious and postinfectious vasculitis can result in stroke; clues for this risk factor include the presence of pharyngitis, sinusitis, bacterial meningitis, chickenpox, pneumonia, HIV, syphilis, or tuberculosis. Cerebral venous thrombosis can also arise due to dehydration; infections of the ears, nose, sinuses, and meninges; and oral estrogen-containing medications.

Mitochondrial encephalomyopathy, lactic acidosis, and stroke-like episodes (MELAS) commonly presents in childhood with stroke syndromes, often accompanied by migraine-like headaches. Cerebral autosomal dominant arteriopathy with subcortical infarcts and leukoencephalopathy (CADASIL) can present (rarely) in the adolescent age group. Migraine can lead to persistent motor aura in the hemiplegic variant which exists in sporadic and familial forms. Partial epilepsy can lead to postictal paralysis (Todd's paralysis), which can also mimic stroke.

Signs and symptoms of stroke are similar in adolescents and adults. This patient had an occlusion of anterior cerebral and middle cerebral branches. Had she presented acutely, tissue plasminogen activator (tPA) and endovascular therapy could have been considered. The cause of this stroke was ultimately found to be a tragic combination of a deep venous thrombosis and PFO. Clearly there are some childhood strokes that could benefit from intravenous thrombolysis. The problem, in addition to the lack of controlled studies of this treatment, is that childhood stroke etiology is more varied than adult stroke, leading to a large number of causes not expected to benefit from tPA. At this time, management of acute stroke in pediatric patients is largely based on hospital-specific guidelines. Additional interventions include good hydration, permissive mild hypertension, and treatment of the underlying mechanism as fast as possible. If seizure is suspected, EEG should be done to attempt to confirm it, and anticonvulsants can be started if there is strong suspicion. Anticoagulants are rarely used. If intracranial pressure (ICP) increases, which can happen in particularly large strokes, as in adults, ICP monitoring can be very helpful in directing measures to reduce pressure, such as hyperosmolar therapy (e.g., mannitol) and even hemicranicetomy. This kind of increase in ICP is fortunately rare in children. Sickle cell disease is managed by repeat blood transfusions.

Diagnostic workup should be thorough and include MRI of the head with DWI and MR venography and MR arteriography of the head and neck in hopes of localizing the pathology. If a dissection is suspected, a fat saturation sequence of the neck vessels should be obtained to increase sensitivity of dissection identification. Echocardiogram is essential for ruling out valvular disease and intracardiac thrombus; this should always be performed with a saline contrast shunt "bubble" study to assess for both intracardiac (e.g., PFO) and extracardiac (e.g., pulmonary AV malformation) shunts. Sickle cell disease should be ruled out, and a coagulation profile should be completed including anticardiolipin, lupus anticoagulant, protein C, protein S, factor V Leiden, fibrinogen, antinuclear antibody, ESR, blood cultures, toxicology screen, urine amino acids, organic acids and homocysteine, lipid panel, basic chemistry panel, blood count, and lactate. Lumbar puncture is indicated if there is concern for CNS infection or vasculitis.

As with anyone with a stroke, secondary prevention and rehab assessment is crucial. A stroke can be emotionally devastating to any patient, but especially to children and adolescents, so careful and thorough explanations and appropriate counseling are both highly important.

KEY POINTS TO REMEMBER

- The causes of stroke in childhood and adolescence include those commonly underlying adult stroke as well as a number of other diseases, including hypercoagulable disorders and vascular anomalies.
- Some conditions can mimic stroke including hemiplegic migraine and postictal paralysis.
- While tPA is probably a useful treatment in many adolescent strokes, the disparity in causation of childhood/adolescent stroke makes it difficult to design a protocol.
- Anticoagulation is only indicated in the acute treatment of stroke in this age group when there is a clear cardiac thromboembolic source or cerebral venous thrombosis.

Further Reading

Amlie-Lefond C, Benedict S, Bernard T, et al. and the International Paediatric Stroke Study Investigators. Thrombolysis in children with arterial ischemic stroke: initial results from the International Paediatric Stroke Study. *Stroke.* 2007;38:485.

Arnold M, Steinlin M, Baumann A, et al. Thrombolysis in childhood stroke: report of 2 cases and review of the literature. *Stroke.* 2009;40:801–807

McGlennan C, Ganesan V. Delays in investigation and management of acute arterial ischaemic stroke in children. *Dev Med Child Neurol.* 2008;50:537–540.

Index

fosphenytoin
    for pain, 125–26
    for status epilepticus, 36t, 38, 39
frontotemporal dementia (FTD), 91, 92–93
functional disorders, 98, 176
functional hemiparesis, 97
functional vital capacity (FVC), 104, 164
fungal meningitis, 48t, 49–50

gabapentin, 144
gadolinium, 119
gastrointestinal bleeding, 112
GBS. *see* Guillain-Barré syndrome
generalized convulsive status epilepticus
        (GCSE), 35, 37f
generalized weakness
    acute, 13
    differential diagnosis, 14, 15t, 16
genetic disorders, 68
giant cell arteritis, 25
give-way weakness, 97, 98–100, 129,
        153, 203
glucocorticoids, 166
glutamic acid decarboxylase (GAD), 69
Guillain-Barré syndrome (GBS)
    acute, 16
    clinical presentation of, 14, 16, 66
    management, 16
    neurophysiological testing for, 15–16
    pathophysiology, 14
    susceptibility for, based on CD4 count,
        84, 84t

Haemophilus influenzae, 48–49
headache
    acute severe, 181–82, 184t
    cluster, 124
    exertional, 31
    International Classification of Headache
        Disorders, 8, 8t, 9t, 126–27, 127t,
        130, 130t
    medication overuse, 131, 132t
    migraine, 129, 179

orgasmic, 31
    in pregnancy, 181–82, 184t
    sentinel, 30t, 31–33
    sudden (thunderclap), 29, 30t
head computed tomography (CT)
    in acute ataxia in child, 200
    before brain biopsy, 88
    in coma with fever, 47–48
    indications, 47–48, 50t, 88, 148,
        170, 200
    before LP, 48, 50t, 170
    single photon emission computed
        tomography (SPECT), 88
    in stroke up to 24 hours, 148
heavy metal intoxication, 14–15
HELLP syndrome, 180
hematoma, 37f, 137f, 138f
hematopoietic cell transplant recipients, 170
hemicrania, paroxysmal, 124
hemiparesis, functional, 97
hemorrhage
    cerebellar, 139
    intracerebral, 135, 137f, 138f
heparin, low-molecular weight
        (LMWH), 113
herpes simplex virus (HSV), 60, 79–80
herpes zoster encephalitis, 93
HIV infection, 14–15, 83
HIV polyradiculoneuropathy, 14–15
HMG-CoA reductase, 106, 107
Hoover's sign, 97, 98–100, 129, 153
hospital-acquired delirium, 41, 44t
hydrocephalus, 140
hydromorphone, 182t
hydroxyzine, 190, 191
hyperactive delirium, 43
hypercalcemia, 14
hypercarbia, 164
hypernatremia, 136–37
hyperosmolality, 136–37
hyperosmolar therapy, 136–37
hyperoxemia, 159–60
hyperperfusion syndrome (HPS), 4, 5

migraine aura
  prolonged, 7, 8*t*
  without headache, 118
migrainous stroke, 8, 9*t*
mild traumatic brain injury (mTBI), 203
Miller Fisher syndrome, 199–200
mitochondrial encephalopathy, lactic
    acidosis, and stroke-like episodes
    syndrome (MELAS), 8–9, 210–11
mononeuritis multiplex, 84, 84*t*
Monroe-Kelli doctrine, 136–37
morphine, 182*t*, 184*t*
Moyamoya disease, 210
multiple sclerosis (MS), 26, 68–69
myasthenia gravis
  clinical presentation, 14–15, 66, 164
  complications, 163
  generalized, 163
  ICPi-associated, 74–76
  management, 75–76
myasthenic crisis, 163
Mycobacterium tuberculosis, 84
mycophenolate mofetil, 166
myelin oligodendrocyte glycoprotein
    antibody (anti-MOG), 68–69
myelitis, 68–69, 74
myelopathy, 16, 65, 67*t*
myocardial infarction, 4, 5, 20
myopathy
  acute, 103
  causes, 104, 105*t*
  inflammatory, 107
  toxic, 107
myositis, 106, 107
myositis antibody panels, 106–7

naloxone trial, 42–43
naproxen, 182*t*
neck flexion strength, 104, 107, 164
neck region nerve injury, postoperative, 4
necrotizing myopathy, immune-mediated,
    106, 107
negative phenomena, 121

neglect, 42–43
Neisseria, 49–50
nerve blocks, occipital, 131, 133
nerve conduction study (NCS), 75, 107
neuralgia
  acute, 123
  definition, 126–27
  primary, 124
  trigeminal, 124–25
neurocardiogenic syncope, 20
neuroleptic malignant syndrome (NMS),
    60–61, 62, 62*t*
neuroleptic medications, 60–61
neuromyelitis optica spectrum disorder
    (NMOSD), 68–69
neuron specific enolase (NSE), 160–61
neuropathic pain, 126–27, 127*t*
neuropathy, painful, 126–27, 127*t*
NIH Stroke Scale (NIHSS), 148
nitrous oxide canisters
    (whippits), 68
nivolumab, 74
NMDA receptors, 92*t*, 93
Nocardia, 84
nonepileptic spells, 175
nonsteroidal anti-inflammatory
    drugs, 181–82

occipital lobe epilepsy, 8–9
occipital nerve blocks, 131, 133
ondansetron, 190
opioids
  avoid use, 132–33
  pregnancy risk, 181–82
optic nerve disease, 24, 26
optic neuritis (ON), 26
orgasmic headache, 31
orthostatic hypotension, 19
overdose
  anticholinergic, 61, 62, 62*t*
  drug, 14, 20, 209
  heavy metal, 14–15
oxcarbazepine, 144

prothrombin complex concentrate (PCC), 138

psychogenic nonepileptic seizures (PNES), 175

psychogenic syncope, 20

psychogenic vertigo, 56

pulmonary embolism, 20

purple-glove syndrome, 38, 125–26

pyridostigmine, 76, 166, 167

pyridoxine (vitamin B6), 38

rabies, 61

raccoon eyes, 204

rescue medications, 131

respiratory distress, 164

respiratory failure
  causes, 164
  differential diagnosis, 165

respiratory function tests, 164

respiratory weakness, 167

retinal artery occlusion, 24–25

retinal detachment, 24

retinal ischemia, 24–25

return to play, 206, 207

reversible cerebral vasoconstriction syndrome (RCVS), 8–9, 30–31, 170, 180

rewarming, 159–60

rhabdomyolysis, 60–61

rivaroxaban (Xarelto), 113, 114*t*, 138

saddle anesthesia, 78

saline, hypertonic, 136–37

Schistosoma, 69

seizures
  causes, 142, 143*t*
  in children, 193
  conditions which mimic, 142
  encephalopathy and, 169
  febrile, 193, 194*t*
  first-time, 141, 143*t*
  generalized, 20, 143–44
  partial (focal), 144

postictal state, 37*f*

prevention of, 145

psychogenic nonepileptic, 175

recurrence, 142–44

risk factors for recurrence, 142–43

subclinical, 38–39

threshold for, 143–44

after transplant, 169

treatment, 38, 39, 139, 142–43

selective serotonin-reuptake inhibitors (SSRI), 177

sensory loss, midline-splitting, 98–100

sensory testing, 42–43

sentinel headache, 30*t*, 31–33

Seroquel, 44

serotonin syndrome (SS), 60, 61–62, 62*t*

shivering control, 159, 161

short-lasting unilateral neuralgiform headache with conjunctival injection and tearing (SUNCT), 124

sickle cell disease, 210, 211–12

sickle cell trait, 210

sick role, 100–1

single photon emission computed tomography (SPECT), 88

sinusitis, sphenoid, 31

skull fracture, 204

sleep-wake cycle, 44, 45

smoking cessation, 121

solid organ transplant recipients, 170

somatic symptom disorder, 101

somatoform disorders, 98

somatosensory evoked potentials (SSEPs), 160–61

spells, nonepileptic, 175

sphenoid sinusitis, 31

spinal cord lesions, 15–16

spinal dural arteriovenous fistula, 68

spontaneous intracranial hypotension, 31

sports injury, adolescent, 203

spot sign, 136

SRP, 106

Staphylococcus, 48–49

trigeminal nerve, 5
trigeminal neuralgia (TN), 124–27
    classification, 126–27, 127*t*
    differential diagnosis, 124, 125*t*
triptans, 182
tuberculosis (TB)
    in cauda equina syndrome, 79–80
    in HIV or AIDS, 84
    susceptibility for, based on CD4 count,
       84, 84*t*
tumors, 92*t*, 93

upper spinal cord lesions, 14

vagus nerve, 5
valproate
    for pain, 131
    for seizures, 144–45
    for status epilepticus, 36*t*, 38, 39
vancomycin, 49
varicella zoster virus (VZV), 60, 79–80, 199
vascular malformations, 68
vasovagal syncope, 20
ventriculostomy, 139
vertebral artery dissection, 8–9, 31, 54
vertebrobasilar transient ischemic
    attack, 8–9
vertigo
    benign positional, 54–55
    causes, 56, 57*t*
    new-onset, 56
    peripheral, 54–55

persistent postural perceptual, 55–56
psychogenic, 56
refractory, 53
treatment, 57–58
vessel imaging, 140. *see also specific
    modalities*
vestibular migraine (VM), 55–56
video-EEG monitoring, 177
viral encephalitis, 60, 61
viral meningitis, 48*t*, 49–51
visual loss, monocular, 23
vitamin B6 (pyridoxine), 38
vitamin K, 138

Wallenberg syndrome, 54
warfarin, 113, 114*t*, 120, 137
weakness
    diaphragmatic, 104
    generalized, 13, 15*t*
    give-way, 97, 98–100, 129, 153,
       203
    neck flexion, 104, 164
    respiratory, 167
    subacute progressive, 14
Wernicke's encephalopathy, 42, 43, 45
whippits (nitrous oxide canisters), 68
white blood cells (WBCs), 142

Xarelto (rivaroxaban), 113, 114*t*

zinc excess, 68
zonisamide, 144–45